Praise for *Anatomy & Yoga*

Ellen Saltonstall's *Anatomy & Yoga* is a clear, comprehensive and beautiful resource for all teachers and serious students of yoga. It has a user-friendly layout, is well illustrated and serves as a great addition to a yoga teacher training course. Each chapter includes a short quiz of the material covered, as well as simple exercises to help with embodied cognition. Saltonstall's fascination and love for her subject shines through on each page, making this an anatomy reference that's engaging, fun and interactive. The book's format make the questions and knowledge jump off the page—in fact, this exploration of anatomy climbs into your body where it belongs. I strongly recommend *Anatomy & Yoga* for anyone who is fascinated with yoga and the human body. **Carrie Owerko, senior certified teacher of Iyengar Yoga, Laban Movement Analyst**

This book should be required reading for all yoga teachers and dedicated students who want to know more about the bodies in which they live and practice. Saltonstall interweaves Tantric philosophy and includes exercises of inquiry to make this book an interactive experience for the reader. This will be a great addition to any yoga library. **Desiree Rumbaugh, internationally acclaimed teacher, author of DVD series *Yoga to the Rescue*, passionate advocate for the transformational power of yoga**

This step-by-step anatomy for yoga book is the best I've seen, with a blend of yogic wisdom and anatomical sophistication. Meticulously detailed but not obscuring the overview, relevant yet profound, the work gracefully combines many elements, like a modern (and ancient) dance. I cannot recommend any other anatomy book as highly as this one, and encourage every yogi, whether practicing for one day or a century, to read it for knowledge and for pleasure. John Karapelou's beautiful pictures are simple (but not too simple), and unlike most anatomical pictures, they are calming. **Loren Fishman MD, B.Phil.,(oxon.) Columbia University**

Anatomy & Yoga is a treasure trove of discovery for anyone interested in exploring the deep intelligence of the body. With compassion, encouragement and humor, Ellen Saltonstall has created a book that makes complexity graspable through explicit diagrams and down-to-earth examples. The book's skillful mix of didactic information coupled with experiential applications will enrich the practice of anyone who teaches yoga or body-mind practices. The wholeness of the body is established as one brilliant system. Inherent in this book is learning that can continue to unfold for a long time and is truly a gift for anyone with a body! **Florence Meleo-Meyer, MS, MA, University of Massachusetts Medical School Center for Mindfulness, Healthcare and Society**

Anatomy & Yoga yokes the rich discernment of the asana to the engineering under the skin, reflecting yogic consciousness while giving it form. Saltonstall's calm, disciplined voice helps the reader visualize and experience anatomy in movement. Illustrations, explanations with examples drawn from asana, and guided experiential learning segments keep both anatomy and yoga vital and immediate.
George Russell, chiropractor, bodyworker, trainer in yoga anatomy, technique and teaching at Kripalu Center for Yoga and Health

Intelligent, clear and inspiring! Reading this book will engage beginners and yoga-nerds alike with the miracle of embodiment. In *Anatomy & Yoga* Saltonstall balances biomechanics brilliantly with philosophy, inspiration and heart from the yoga tradition. The study questions and exercises presented with each section are accessible and effective. They will provide a reliable way for newer students of anatomy to directly experience the information. I have accumulated 26 anatomy texts and nearly as many anatomy apps and webinars. I am not exaggerating to say that # 27 – *Anatomy & Yoga* - is definitely the one I will be using in my yoga teacher trainings from now on. **Karen Sprute-Francovich, M.A., certified Anusara Yoga teacher & teacher trainer, co-chair Anusara Curriculum Committee**

Anatomy & Yoga is a brilliant work of clarity, elegance, simplicity and functionality. I love it! Normally, learning anatomy is dry and boring. But through Ellen Saltonstall's exquisite organizational skills and precision, I found myself devouring the pages. What's unique about this anatomy book is how the information is so easily assimilated. Based on excellent, therapeutic alignment techniques, each chapter concludes with a summarizing quiz. I plan to use this book in my professional training courses. This book is a gift to all yoga teachers. **Todd Norian, founder of Ashaya Yoga®**

Ellen Saltonstall's book is destined to become standard reading for yoga teacher trainings. She has found a way to balance depth and sophistication with clarity and utility. If this is the first biomechanical book you read, you'll walk away with a real understanding of how the body moves, and studied professionals will find her presentation both thought-provoking and illuminating.
Ross Rayburn, international yoga teacher

Ellen Saltonstall's writing demonstrates her many years of knowledge and experience as a master therapeutic yoga teacher. This is a rare find: an anatomy book that can speak specifically to yoga anatomy and yoga therapeutics in an accessible and holistic way. While maintaining the clear anatomical approach, Ellen succeeds in showing the reader how deeply connected our anatomical system is. This offering is a powerful and functional tool for yoga teachers looking for clarity, connection and applicable teachings. **Tara Glazier, owner/founder of Abhaya Yoga**

In *Anatomy & Yoga*, Ellen Saltonstall generously offers her wisdom on body mechanics from decades of dance, yoga and bodywork. The book is a succinct, interactive guide for yoga practitioners and teachers of any level to deepen their understanding of functional anatomy in the context of yoga practice and healthy movement. The author expertly takes an often-overwhelming subject and makes it fun and approachable with defined anatomical terminology, simple explanations, clear illustrations, exercises and practical information immediately applicable to your practice. The book is organized for the reader to focus on basic functions, or to go deeper in their body knowledge. There are interactive examples to explore in your own body, and study questions at the end of each chapter for maximum absorption of material. I highly recommend this book to all yoga practitioners, yoga teachers and yoga therapists. **Kelly Haas, Integrative Yoga teacher, yoga therapist, certified Anusara Yoga teacher**

With this book, all levels of yoga practitioners have a welcome storehouse of information about the connectedness of all parts of the body in yoga practice. Beginners will find the basics about how the human body is constructed and how it operates, and experienced practitioners and teachers will find interesting and thought-provoking details regarding the coordination of the parts with the whole.
Mel Robin, certified Iyengar Yoga teacher and author of *A Physiological Handbook for Teachers of Yogasana*

This book is a rare find. It is easy to read, very clear, and an incredible resource for yoga students and teachers. It is also an invaluable tool for teacher trainings, with many examples of how to experience the workings of the body in asana practice. With Saltonstall's vast knowledge and dedication to the art of anatomy and yoga, she presents a comprehensive map of the human body. **Jim Bernaert, certified Anusara Yoga teacher and teacher trainer**

Finally! A comprehensive anatomy book especially for yoga students. Ellen Saltonstall's clear and detailed explanations of the anatomy and biomechanics of movement specifically tailored to yoga practitioners are a gift to teachers and students alike. As a teacher, teacher trainer and student of yoga, I'll refer to this book for years to come. **Barrie Risman, co-director World Spine Care Yoga Project, Montreal, Canada**

Wonderfully concise and clear, *Anatomy & Yoga* is sure to become one of the most-used guides for yoga teachers and students alike. Ellen Saltonstall has teased out the most important concepts one needs to know when applying the complex subject of anatomy to asana practice and presented them in a format that is clear and easy to follow. The book brilliantly illustrates the interrelationships between individual parts of the body in a way that encourages critical thinking, fostering a holistic understanding of anatomy that goes well beyond memorizing names and actions of muscles. Practice suggestions provide the reader with the opportunity to immediately apply the information through movement, touch, and feeling on one's own or another's body. As an anatomy teacher for yoga teachers in training, I will be requiring *Anatomy & Yoga* as the main reference book for my classes. **Kristine Whittle, yoga teacher trainer, LMT, assistant director, Control Group Productions**

Ellen Saltonstall's new book, *Anatomy & Yoga*, is comprehensive and easy to read, and it contains a full exploration of the amazing human body and its functioning for a healthy and balanced yoga practice. Saltonstall combines her immense wonder of the body and life-long movement study into this one gem of a book. I will definitely be using this book for the anatomy portion of future teacher training programs. **Julie Dohrman, yoga instructor, teacher trainer and founder of Shaktiyoga New York**

Ellen Saltonstall is celebrated for her ability to bring anatomy to a level that all students can understand and apply to their yoga practices. This book is a must for teachers, teacher trainings, students and anyone else who is interested in knowing more about their bodies as they relate to yoga or other movement modalities. Well written with excellent graphics! **Karen Rider, certified yoga instructor, teacher trainer**

This book is a masterful, user-friendly guide for any serious student/teacher of yoga. The text and illustrations flow beautifully together to engage and inspire the reader. I would certainly recommend this book to any of my students. **Kali Morse, director, Teacher Trainings Integral Yoga Institute**

ANATOMY & YOGA

Also by Ellen Saltonstall

Yoga for Arthritis
Co-authored with Dr. Loren Fishman
WW Norton, 2008

Yoga for Osteoporosis
Co-authored with Dr. Loren Fishman
WW Norton, 2010

ANATOMY & YOGA

A Guide for Teachers and Students

Ellen Saltonstall

Illustrated by John Karapelou and Liem Nguyen

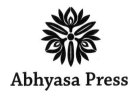

Abhyasa Press

ANATOMY AND YOGA
A Guide for Teachers and Students
Text © 2016 by Ellen Saltonstall
Illustrations © 2016 by John Karapelou or Liem Nguyen, as indicated

The information in this book is offered solely for the purpose of education. For all health or medical issues, consult a qualified healthcare provider. It is also advisable to practice yoga with the guidance of a qualified instructor.

Abhyasa Press
17 E 16th Street #5
New York, NY 10003
info@abhyasapress.com

Cover illustration by Liem Nguyen
Interior illustrations by John Karapelou and Liem Nguyen
Cover design by Molly Heron
Indexing by Sheilagh and Elspeth Simpson

Publisher's Cataloging-In-Publication Data
(Prepared by The Donohue Group, Inc.)

Names: Saltonstall, Ellen. | Karapelou, John W., illustrator. | Nguyen, Liem, illustrator.
Title: Anatomy and yoga : a guide for teachers and students / Ellen Saltonstall ; illustrations by John Karapelou and Liem Nguyen.
Description: New York, NY : Abhyasa Press, [2016] | Includes index.
Identifiers: ISBN 978-0-9978561-0-1 | ISBN 978-0-9978561-1-8 (ePub) | ISBN 978-0-9978561-2-5 (Mobipocket)
Subjects: LCSH: Human anatomy--Handbooks, manuals, etc. | Yoga--Physiological aspects--Handbooks, manuals, etc.
Classification: LCC QM28 .S25 2016 (print) | LCC QM28 (ebook) | DDC 611--dc23

10 9 8 7 6 5 4 3 2 1

Printed in the United States of America on paper that is certified by the Forest Stewardship Council and the Rainforest Alliance

Table of Contents

Acknowledgments

Thanks to my parents for their unconditional support of me and for the values of diligence, generosity, persistence and honesty by which they lived. From decades of my professional life spent in dance, yoga and bodywork, I am grateful to many teachers, notably Elaine Summers, Merce Cunningham, Anahid Sofian, John Friend, Mary Dunn and Carrie Owerko—their joy in movement was and is contagious. Thanks to the anatomy teachers whose wisdom has inspired me: Dorothy Vislocky, Irene Dowd and Thomas Myers. My students and clients have supported me, challenged me and fueled me to continue learning. A project with Martin Kirk was the impetus to produce this text, and I value our discussions over six years of collaboration. Several friends and colleagues took the time to read early drafts of this text and gave me valuable feedback; thanks to Dr. Loren Fishman, David Fink, Susan Genis, Jim Bernaert, Ruthie Bernaert, Jayendra Hanley and Dina Ghen. Thanks to Molly Heron (yoga teacher and designer) for her keen eye and generous spirit in producing the cover design. Illustrators John Karapelou and Liem Nguyen have enriched this book with their excellent artwork. Special thanks to my family for their constancy and support.

Introduction

Welcome to the study of anatomy: the study of your own body, the body you live in, the body you practice yoga in. If you're reading this book, you probably have some curiosity about what happens under your skin as you practice yoga. You may want to understand how the joints and muscles and connective tissues all work together to enable you to do your asana practice. You may want to avoid injuries with the help of that understanding. If you're a teacher, you hopefully want to help your students practice safely and intelligently, respecting the biomechanics of the body while also having fun with the practice. A bit of knowledge goes a long way in empowering your students to receive all the benefits that yoga has to offer.

With more and more people coming to yoga for good health, it's increasingly important for teachers to be well informed about the body. Students rely on teachers to guide them, and it's a big responsibility to be the temporary caretaker of your students while they are in class. We need to understand what demands the practice is making and what actions will produce the best results. Your anatomy knowledge can be invisible to the students, but it will give you essential confidence in what you are saying. As a teacher, you don't need to call out the names of muscles ("Now, fire your flexor digitorum profundus!"), but it's good to know why the instruction to "press your fingertips down" will be beneficial for your students, to give just one example.

Human anatomy is a huge body of knowledge, and one that is growing constantly. Researchers are not discovering new muscles, but we are recognizing more ways in which the body's intelligence connects all of our separate parts into one whole. As we study the body, we identify the parts, but we also consider the interrelationships. How do the feet determine the health of the lower back? How does the carriage of your head influence the entire body? These connections will be part of the discussion in this text.

Don't be dismayed by the abundance of terms and details. Just start from wherever you are in your understanding, and build on it one step at a time. Read one chapter at a time, applying it to your own body, and the information will settle in. The text offers many opportunities to apply the information in the moment, with your own body or with a fellow student. Moving, touching and feeling is the best way to learn. When there are many different muscles in a certain area of the body, I've indicated which ones to start with for those just beginning their study. Start with those smaller bites, then add on others when you are ready. Little by little, the pieces will fit together for a more complete picture of your body in yoga. This text can serve as a guide and reference for your ongoing study. Your yoga practice can be the laboratory for flashes of insight.

I began my study of anatomy many years ago as a dancer and massage therapist. Very soon I wanted to go beyond the basics of naming the muscles and joints to figure out why my friends and clients had various injuries and chronic pain. And, of course, I wanted to understand my own unique body patterns and how they played out in my movement experiences. When I began to practice yoga, I realized its huge potential for bringing strength, openness and balance to the body and the mind. Now as I train other yoga teachers, my hope is that this body of knowledge becomes as familiar as moving into Downward-Facing Dog.

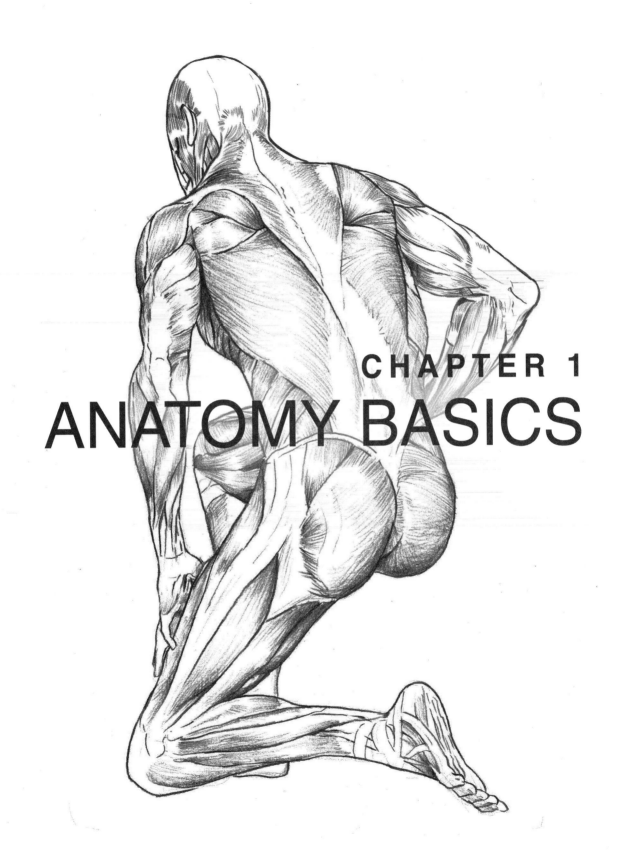

CHAPTER 1
ANATOMY BASICS

Tantra is a philosophy, a view of humanity and a spiritual path that honors sacredness in all aspects of human life. Tantra developed in India in the ninth century, building on many other existing spiritual traditions. In Tantric philosophy the human body is considered to be an expression of the highest consciousness in condensed form. A Tantric yoga practice includes caring for this body so that it can be a vibrantly healthy vehicle for our spiritual journey. When we are healthy, it's easier to remember our highest self. A yoga practice helps us to celebrate life with a strong body, a sharp mind and a soft heart.

A movement in yoga practice is not just a means to an end; it is the recognition of all parts of the body as manifestations of energy. All the separate elements of the body—the bones, muscles, breath, organs and mind—are completely interwoven and affect each other in every moment of our lives, including in every moment of our asana practice. In order to understand these elements of the body more deeply and fully, we separate the elements, and we identify and study them, knowing that each is part of a greater whole. Awareness and knowledge of these physical structures will help to clarify the alignment principles we follow in yoga, to deepen our experience of asana practice and to enrich our celebration of life.

For those entering the study of anatomy for the first time, it is like learning a new language. Many terms may be unfamiliar to you, and you will be visualizing what is normally unseen inside the body. Be patient with yourself as you begin this study! There will be frequent examples and exercises for you to apply these concepts to your own body in order to make it more experiential. Each group of muscles will be divided into subgroups to give you a step-by-step sequence to follow in your study. Beginners can learn just the most important muscles, and as you're ready, you can add to your bank of vocabulary and knowledge.

The purpose of this chapter is to define terms that will recur as we move along in the study process and to provide some basic information about the types of tissues in the body that affect our yoga practice.

Anatomical Neutral Position

In order to describe the location and function of different structures in the body, anatomists have agreed upon a neutral starting position as a reference. The universally accepted **anatomical neutral position** is standing erect with the legs straight, feet roughly pointing forward and hip joint–width apart, and the arms hanging by the sides with the palms facing forward. Note that this is not the same as *Tadasana* (Mountain Pose), in which the palms face in toward the sides. All joint movements, muscle locations and actions can be identified and described relative to this starting position. For instance, hip flexion and extension are defined in reference to this particular neutral position; hip flexion brings your leg to the front, and hip extension takes your leg behind you. Even when we analyze a pose that may be far flung from this position (such as an inversion, deep twist or both), we use this same position as a reference to determine what the joints and muscles are doing.

The Spatial Planes

There are three basic spatial planes within which any movement occurs: **frontal, sagittal and transverse** (see Figure 1.1). Understanding the planes is helpful as we examine our movements and the requirements of the joints in doing each one. When we swing our arms to the sides and up, as in jumping jacks, we are tracing the shape of the **frontal** (also called the **coronal**) plane. It divides the body into a front half and a back half. There are two types of movements that occur in this plane. One is **adduction**, moving a limb closer to or across the midline, such as crossing the legs and arms in *Garudasana* (Eagle Pose). The other is **abduction**, moving a limb away from the midline. We abduct both the legs and arms in *Virabhadrasana II* (Warrior Pose) and the legs in *Upavishtha Konasana* (Seated Wide Angle Pose).

The **sagittal** plane divides the body into left and right sides. When we walk and swing our arms forward and back, the legs and arms move in a sagittal plane. *Surya Namaskar* (Sun Salutation) occurs in the sagittal plane. The mid-sagittal plane is the centerline of the body between right and left. It is also called the median plane. Forward and backward bending poses such as *Adho Mukha Shvanasana* (Downward-Facing Dog Pose) and *Virabhadrasana I* exemplify this plane.

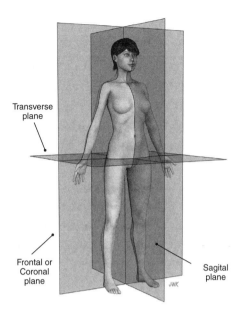

Figure 1.1 *Three spatial planes*

The movements in the sagittal plane are **flexion**, defined as shortening the joint angle at the front of the body, and **extension**, defined as shortening the joint angle at the back of the body. For instance, if you stand in the anatomical neutral position and bend your elbow as if to bring a cup to your mouth to drink, you are performing flexion of both the elbow and the shoulder joints. Reaching your arm behind you to put on a coat is an example of extension of the shoulder joint. Forward-bending poses and back-bending poses move in the sagittal plane.

The toes, knees and ankles are exceptions to this rule. If you bend one knee to take your foot behind you, that is called knee flexion even though it shortens the angle of your knee joint in the back instead of the front. The return from flexion is considered to be extension. Curling your toes under is flexion; lifting them up is extension. The specific movement terms for the ankle joint are **dorsiflexion** (drawing the top of your foot up toward the front of your shin, as in Adho Mukha Shvanasana) and **plantar flexion** (pressing your toes away from your shin, aka "pointing" the foot, as in *Virasana* (Hero Pose). One way to remember these distinctions is that dorsiflexion moves toward the dorsal (top) side of the foot (as in the dorsal fin of a shark, which is on top). Plantar flexion moves toward the bottom of the foot where the plantar fascia is, where you "plant" your foot on the ground.

The third plane, the **transverse** plane, is horizontal like a tabletop and divides the body into upper and lower segments. When we move in this plane, we rotate around an axis. All twisting poses move through this plane in some way. Two types of rotation are possible with the arms or the legs in this plane: lateral rotation is defined as turning a point on the front of the limb away from the midline, and medial rotation is turning toward the midline. If you touch the front of your thigh with your finger, for instance, medial rotation of your thigh will move your finger toward the midline of your body, and lateral rotation will move it away from your midline.

Directional Terms

Again for the sake of clarity, anatomists have agreed on terms that describe location by defining the relative position of one body part to another. These terms come in pairs:

superior: above
inferior: below

medial: closer to the midline
lateral: farther from the midline

anterior: toward the front
posterior: toward the back

superficial: toward the surface
deep: farther from the surface

proximal: closer to the origin of a limb or the center of the trunk
distal: farther from the origin of a limb or the center of the trunk

intermediate: between the two extremes of any of these pairs of opposites

Examples:

The head is superior to the pelvis.

The arm is lateral to the spine.

The navel is anterior to the spine.

The skin is superficial to the femur bone.

The fingers are distal to the elbow.

The collarbones are intermediate to the shoulder joints and the breastbone.

It is important to recognize how the use of some of these terms in everyday language differs from their anatomical definitions. For instance, notice how these statements have different meanings in anatomical language versus everyday language:

- "The head is superior to the heart." In anatomical language this means that the head is spatially above the heart, but in everyday language you might think it means that the head is more valuable or important than the heart.

- "Extend your arms" in everyday language could mean a variety of things. In anatomical language, the word "extend" would refer to the specific action at the shoulder joint when your arms move behind you.

From One Cell to Endless Diversity

The development of a human body from one fertilized egg cell is nothing short of a miracle. Through millions of cell divisions, the body grows into a structure of such complexity and subtlety that modern science has yet to understand all its functions. Each cell, and each group of cells that form tissues, has a particular role to play and its own characteristics. There is an intelligence and order underlying the complexity of this development from the very moment we are conceived. Stem cells, which can become any type of cell, develop in particular ways in response to their physical and chemical environment. They grow in ways that prepare them for the structure and function of the body tissue they inhabit. Cells become specialized and group together to form tissues. Tissues combine to form organs, and organs are grouped together into systems. Scientists can now participate in the creative power of the body's intelligence. By creating an environment that mimics a particular body tissue, they "invite" stem cells to develop with a specific structure for a specific function.

Types of Tissues

The four primary types of tissue in the body are epithelial, muscle, nerve and connective tissue. All types are involved with our practice of yoga, especially connective tissue, which is the most abundant type of tissue in the body.

Epithelial Tissue

Epithelial tissue includes the skin, the linings of organs, and the glands. Glands are organs that secrete substances into specialized ducts or into the bloodstream. Epithelial tissue has four functions:

- **Protection** (e.g., the skin)
- **Absorption** (e.g., the lining of the digestive tract)
- **Filtration** (e.g., the kidneys)
- **Secretion** (e.g. the mucous membranes, sweat glands, endocrine glands)

Muscle Tissue

The specialty of muscle tissue is to contract or shorten to produce movement of the bones, the organs or the heart. There are three types of muscles:

- **Skeletal** or **striated muscle** moves the bones and is voluntarily controlled. All the muscles that we use to bend our joints and move our limbs into yoga poses are skeletal muscles.

- **Smooth** or **visceral muscle** moves the internal organs and the walls of blood vessels and does not require our voluntary control. For example, when we experience stress, the blood vessels receive a signal from the nervous system to reduce blood supply to the digestive system and increase blood supply to the skeletal muscles so that we can escape danger. The smooth muscles in the vessel walls either constrict or relax the vessels to route the blood to where it is most needed.

- **Cardiac muscle** is found only in the heart and operates this vital organ as a constant pump.

Skeletal muscles come in many different shapes and sizes. Some are spindle shaped, others broad and more rectangular, others fan shaped. Each muscle has three parts:

- A **belly**, where the contracting fibers are.
- An **origin**, where the muscle begins.
- An **insertion**, where the muscle attaches.

The attachments are generally tendons, although there are exceptions to that rule. The origin is generally considered to be the attachment on the more stable bone, the insertion on the more mobile bone. In most cases, the more stable bone will be the most proximal one, close to the core of the body. When the fibers contract toward the middle, shortening the muscle, this is called concentric contraction ("con" means "to" or "with," meaning that it goes toward the center.)

There are times when we move the origin toward the insertion instead of moving the insertion toward the origin. Here's an example: The origin of the pectoralis major muscle (on the front chest) is on the sternum, and its insertion is on the arm. Generally, the pectoralis major moves the arm across the front of the body (adduction) with the trunk staying still, such as in a forehand stroke in tennis or when the hands come into *Anjali Mudra* (Prayer Position). However, in yoga we often reverse this situation and do a movement that moves the origin toward the insertion. For example, when the hand is weight bearing on the floor in *Vasishthasana* (Side Plank Pose), we use the pectoralis major muscle to turn back to Plank Pose, onto two hands. In this case, the insertion at the periphery (the arm) is the stable part, and the origin (the chest) moves toward it. Another example is turning the torso toward the extended leg in *Janushirshasana* (Head to Knee Pose). We activate the adductor muscles not to move the leg (the distal attachment of the adductor muscles), but to move the pelvis (the proximal attachment of the adductor muscles). Currently, anatomists tend to refer to the places that muscles connect to bones simply as the "proximal" and "distal" attachments, rather than as the "origin" and "insertion." I mention these terms here because they are found in many anatomy books.

Muscles can also contract and lengthen at the same time, which is called **eccentric contraction** ("e" refers to movement away or out, as in "exit" or "egress"). A yoga example of this is moving into Virabhadrasana II, when you bend the knee to the proper alignment directly over your ankle. The quadriceps muscles are lengthening since the knee is bending, but they are also contracting to control the rate of bending. If they released totally, we'd fall down! Another example is lowering the arms slowly in order to move in tandem with the breath; our muscle contraction slows the pace of movement. Eccentric contraction is usually done while resisting another force, such as gravity.

Concentric and eccentric contraction are both types of **isotonic contractions**, meaning that the length of the muscle changes while the tone may not ("iso" means "one" or "same"). Eccentric contraction generally will strengthen the muscles more quickly. Have you noticed how much work the quadriceps muscles do when you climb down a mountain? Not only are your thighs tired from the climb up, but the eccentric contraction required on the way down is hard work as well! When the weight goes onto the forward foot, the quadriceps work to control the rate of descent in an eccentric contraction.

Once you arrive at the bent-knee position in Virabhadrasana II, you hold it with **isometric contraction**, in which the muscle does not change length while contracting ("iso" means "the same," and "metric" means "length"). This type of contraction is also done while resisting another force, which could be gravity or another limb of the body. For example, the arm and the leg pressing against each other in *Ardha Matsyendrasana* (Seated Lord of the Fishes Twist) create isometric contractions in the muscles of both limbs. Much of the muscular effort we use in yoga is isometric contraction.

A muscle that produces a given action is called the **agonist** or **prime mover**, and the muscle that produces the opposite action is called the **antagonist** or **opposing muscle**. For example, when you bend your elbow, the biceps at the front of the arm is the agonist, and the triceps in the back (whose job is to straighten the elbow) is the antagonist. Here are some pairs of agonists and antagonists:

Muscle Pair: Biceps and triceps
Function: Bending and straightening the elbow

Muscle Pair: Hamstrings and quadriceps
Function: Bending and straightening the knee

Muscle Pair: Gastrocnemius and tibialis anterior
Function: Plantar flexion and dorsiflexion of the ankle

Muscle Pair: Rectus abdominis and erector spinae
Function: Flexing and extending the spine

Muscle Pair: Supinators and pronators of the forearm
Function: Turning the palm up and down

Some muscles are large enough to be their own antagonists. The deltoid, for example, has three sections spanning the top of the shoulder. The anterior section pulls the arm forward, whereas the posterior section pulls the arm back.

There are also **synergists** that assist the agonist, and **stabilizers** that work to hold a neighboring part of the body steady in order to allow the agonist to have more power. For example, the gastrocnemius and the soleus muscles are synergists in plantar flexion, or pointing the foot. The abdominals and the spinal extensors both serve as stabilizers for the pelvis when hip flexion occurs, as in *Supta Padangushtasana* (Reclining Hamstring Stretch).

In yoga, as in any complex movement activity, we use muscles in an intricate teamwork, a constantly shifting yet identifiable pattern of cooperation toward the goals of stability and freedom. In other words, using an agonist and its antagonist muscle simultaneously is exactly what can lead to a balanced and well-supported action in yoga. Often, a muscle is being stretched while still acting as a stabilizer, for example:

- The adductor muscles on the inner thighs are stretched in *Utthita Trikonasana* (Triangle Pose), yet they are also acting to stabilize our stance.

- The abdominal muscles are stretched as antagonists in a deep backbend such as *Urdhva Dhanurasana* (Upward-Facing Bow Pose), yet they are also needed as stabilizers for the lower back.

- The outer hip muscles are strongly stretched in Garudasana, yet they are needed for balance as well.

The tone of a muscle is usually defined as the tension present when the muscle is resting. We can call this "passive tone," whereas "active tone" is the tension present in the muscle when it is active. The tone reflects the pattern of use in that muscle (more use will result in higher tone) and is also determined by individual body chemistry.

Factors to Look for When Studying Muscles

As you study the muscles, I suggest you keep the following factors in mind, which will help you to understand the biomechanics of each body part more fully.

- What are the exact attachment points of the muscle? This will tell you the direction of each muscle's pull on the bones.

- Does the muscle cross one joint (monoarticular) or more than one joint (polyarticular)? The forces at work in polyarticular muscles will be more complex than in monoarticular muscles.

- What is the shape of the joint? This will determine what movement is possible for the muscles to create. Ball-and-socket joints (such as the shoulder) have the biggest range of motion, whereas flatter joints (such as the knee) have less range.

- What is the muscle's relationship to gravity in the position or movement you are considering?

- How is the muscle's potential for contraction or stretch being influenced by its relationships to other structures and its place in the bigger picture of the fascial web? (See more about the fascial web in the section below on connective tissue.)

Nerve Tissue

Nerve tissue conveys electrochemical messages between the brain and every part of the body at a miraculous speed. Some nerves report to us about sensation and body position (called **afferent** nerves, meaning that they bring messages back to the brain from the outside world), while others (called **efferent** nerves), direct movement or other functions by sending messages out from the brain to the muscles or organs. The **neuron** is the basic cell type of this tissue; some neurons are up to three feet long.

Connective Tissue

Connective tissue is the most abundant type of tissue in the body and the most varied in its texture, shape and function. Some types of connective tissue are liquid, such as blood and lymph. Others are soft padding materials such as areolar tissue and adipose tissue (also known as fat), and harder padding tissues like cartilage. Bones are connective tissue, and due to their high mineral content, bones are solid enough to provide support

(in our spine, arms and legs) and protection (in our skull). There are also many types of semi-pliable connective tissues such as ligaments, tendons and fascia whose functions of connection and force transmission are essential for coordinating our movements.

Each of these different types of connective tissue has a matrix and cellular components that determine its characteristic texture. The matrix can be very hard, semi-soft, very soft or liquid. Within this matrix is a combination of several types of cells. In the connective tissues such as bones, tendons, ligaments and fascia, these cells are composed of collagen, elastin and reticulin. The proportion of these components will vary according to the function of the tissue. Tissues that function more as support, such as bone and cartilage, will have more collagen, whereas tissues that need to withstand more stretching, such as ligaments and tendons, will have more elastin. Whereas elastin fibers can stretch up to 200 percent of their original length without damage (useful in the walls of blood vessels, for instance), collagen fibers can stretch only 10 percent (useful for stability in the bones and cartilage). Reticulin fibers are a precursor to collagen and are less abundant in the body.

In terms of function, we can summarize by saying that connective tissue protects, transports, supports, connects, separates and organizes other tissues in the body. That's versatility! In this section we will address the forms of connective tissue most involved with movement and yoga.

Bones

We may think of our bones as being hard and unbendable, because the examples we see are either from cadavers or made from hard plastic. In reality, live bone is a dynamic structure full of cellular activity. Bones are constantly being remodeled, and they serve as reservoirs for fat and minerals and as factories for the production of blood cells.

The defining characteristic of bone tissue is its combination of lightness and strength. It has the highest proportion of minerals of any of the connective tissues (70 percent), and although it is firm and strong, it can also stretch a small amount. Its structure allows for both compressive and tensile stress, that is, the types of stress caused by both weight bearing and the pull from muscles as we move. Our bones serve as protection and support for our vital organs, as weight-bearing support and as leverage for the variety of movements we can perform.

The skeleton

The adult human skeleton is composed of 206 bones and is generally divided into two portions: the **axial skeleton** (80 bones of the skull, spine and ribs) and the **appendicular skeleton** (126 bones of the pelvic girdle, the shoulder girdle, and the arms and legs). We can think of the axial skeleton as our core support and the appendicular skeleton as the means by which we connect to the world around us.

Joints

Where two bones meet, a joint is formed. There are three types of joints: **diarthoses** (in Greek, *di* means "two" and *arthro* means "joint"), which move freely (many joints that we will discuss come into this category, including hips, shoulders, elbows and knees); **amphiarthroses**, which move somewhat (e.g., intervertebral joints of the spine and pubic symphysis); and **synarthroses**, which move very little if at all (e.g., the sutures between the skull bones, and between the tibia and fibula in the lower leg).

In the category of freely movable joints, or diarthrotic joints, there are many shapes and many types of movements possible. This list illustrates the diversity of joint types, and you can see them illustrated in Figure 1.2:

- Ball-and-socket, or spheroidal: This type of joint, exemplified by the hips and shoulders, offers the widest range of movements in all planes.

- Condyloid, or ellipsoid: This is the rounded surface of one bone fitting inside a shallow basin-shaped concavity in the other bone. An example is the joint between the radius and the carpal bones at the wrist, and the joints between the base of each finger and its metacarpal bone in the palm. Movement is in two planes here as well (flexion, extension, adduction and abduction). With this type of joint, we can also perform circumduction, which is a sequential combination of these four movements, tracing a circle.

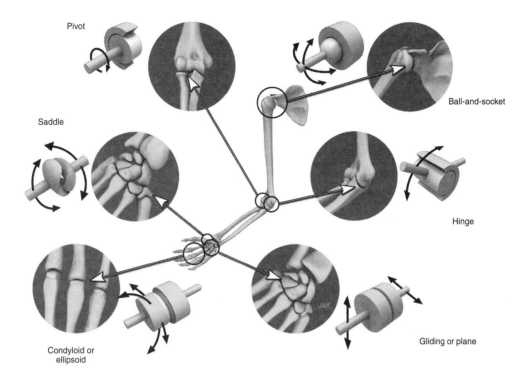

Figure 1.2 *Joint types*

- Saddle: This type of joint resembles two curved surfaces fitting together, like a person sitting on a saddle. One example is the carpometacarpal joint at the base of the thumb. Movement is in two planes: forward and back, and side to side.

- Hinge: Movement is in one plane only, as in the knee, ankle and elbow. The folding and unfolding of flexion and extension are performed at hinge joints.

- Pivot: This joint type allows for rotation, as in the atlas-axis joint between the top two vertebrae of the spine, and the portion of the elbow joint that allows the forearm to rotate.

- Gliding, or plane: Both surfaces of this type of joint are more flat and allow for limited movement. Examples are the joints in the carpals (wrist) and tarsals (feet) between the small irregular-shaped bones there. Another example is the joints between the facet surfaces of the vertebrae.

All diarthrotic joints have what is called a **synovial capsule** ("synovial" means "egg-like") surrounding the joint, within which the lubricating and nourishing **synovial fluid** is secreted. The **synovial membrane** on the inside of the capsule secretes nutrients that feed the cartilage covering the bones. The inside of the joint gets a constant bath of lubrication and sustenance aided by our movement, which helps to keep the bones and cartilage healthy. In our yoga practice we move the joints through a wide range of movements, pumping the synovial fluid optimally throughout the joint space.

Cartilage

Cartilage is a type of connective tissue that is more flexible than bone. Like bone, cartilage is tough enough to withstand both compressive and tensile forces. Unlike bone, however, cartilage does not have its own blood supply and depends on neighboring tissues for its nutrition. There are three types of cartilage:

- Hyaline cartilage covers the ends of bones inside all joints. It is a glossy, smooth tissue, hard enough to protect the bones from the friction of rubbing against each other, yet malleable enough to withstand that pressure without damage. When we move our joints through their respective ranges of motion, our movement facilitates distribution of nutrients to this cartilage.

- Fibrocartilage has more flexibility than hyaline cartilage. It is found in the intervertebral discs, the meniscus of the knee, most joint capsules, the connection of the ribs into the sternum and the joint between the two pubic bones. Its specialty is shock absorption.

- Elastic cartilage is found in parts of the body that need to move even more yet maintain their shape, such as the earlobe and the epiglottis in the throat.

Ligaments

Ligaments connect bone to bone, providing essential structural stability to the joints as we move. They are made up of rope-like strands of collagen-predominant material, which join directly into the coverings of the bones. Ligaments vary in their ability to stretch (depending upon the amount of elastin they contain) and yet maintain the integrity of the structures they are connecting.

For example, the ligaments of the knee do not stretch very much at all without tearing, yet the ligament at the back of the neck elongates up to 200 percent of its original length, allowing us to do poses like *Sarvangasana* (Shoulder Stand), which requires extensive flexion of the cervical spine.

Ligaments tend to be slow in healing when injured, because of poor blood supply. Overstretching ligaments is problematic because it will destabilize the joints. Caution is especially important during pregnancy, when the hormone relaxin is circulating through the body to help the pelvis expand and accommodate the growing fetus.

Individuals vary greatly in their inborn ligament flexibility: some are more mobile, and some are more stiff. On one end of the spectrum, those who can do advanced yoga poses fairly easily were probably born with ligaments long enough to allow a large range of motions in the joints. However, on this same end of the scale, some people who have very lax ligaments cannot retain sufficient stability in their joints. This condition is so common that the medical profession has given it a name: **hypermobility syndrome**, defined as joint laxity with musculoskeletal complaints. In the practice of yoga, students can protect the ligaments from overstretching by building specific muscular strength around the joints. The partial contraction of a muscle that is stretching gives the signal along the entire fascial chain (see the next page in discussion of fascia) to create stability. This contraction-while-stretching also educates the muscles to be resilient in finding the appropriate level of tone for the complex activities of daily life and sports.

On the other end of the spectrum are those yoga students for whom hours and years of stretching result in only minimal freedom in the joints because their ligaments are constructed with less elastin. These students can focus more on flexibility by expanding out from the center in each pose and by practicing diligently to gradually increase their range of motion.

Tendons

Tendons connect muscles to either bones or other connective tissue. Their structure is a beautiful illustration of nature's efficiency and elegance as it transforms into its manifest forms. The connective tissue surrounding a muscle becomes a fibrous tendon at each end by virtue of changes in its composition, and then morphs directly into the coating of the bone or the fascia to which it attaches in a seamless transition. Surprisingly, tendons have a smaller proportion of elastin fibers than ligaments, meaning that they do not readily return to their original length after being stretched.

Although many tendons are rope-like in shape, which makes it easier for them to fit into small joint spaces, some tendons are broad and flat; these are called **aponeuroses**. One example of this type of tendon is the **thoracolumbar aponeurosis** (see Figure 1.3c), the inferior (lower) attachment of the large latissimus dorsi muscle at the back of the waist. In this case the muscle connects to the broad tendon, which is then anchored to the bone.

Bursae and scar tissue

Though not technically considered to be connective tissue, these two structures deserve mention in our discussion because of their importance in studying movement.

Bursae are small fluid-filled sacs that serve as cushions in places where tendons must slide over bony projections. They help prevent friction near the joints, but they can become inflamed when tight muscles produce too much compression close to the joints. Some examples of places where the bursae are located include under the **acromion** of the shoulder, in several places near the kneecap (see Figure 5.4), and between the tendons of the buttocks muscles and the **greater trochanter** of the femur, a bony prominence you can feel at the side of your hip.

Scar tissue is what grows to heal any injury involving a tear or fracture of tissue. Its function is to connect the edges of a wound. We associate scar tissue with the tough, unpigmented skin that grows to heal over a cut or scrape on the surface of the skin, but it also grows under the skin. This healing process is another of nature's miracles: the body recognizes where healing is needed, sends the raw materials to the site very quickly and does the repair. Scar tissue covers and reconnects the area of injury so that healing can take place, after which the scar tissue is integrated into the surrounding tissue. Aggressive yoga or bodywork on a recent injury site could compromise or slow down the process of healing, so it is advisable to allow time for healing after a tear or fracture before resuming a strong yoga practice. The duration of time needed for healing depends on the degree and location of the injury.

Muscle tears can occur during our yoga practice if we work too fast without warming up, if we work beyond our capacity or if we work in poor alignment. The formation of scar tissue is helpful because it provides quick protection when there has been an injury. However, scar tissue is also problematic in that it never has the same level of flexibility and blood supply as the original tissue. It will be tougher and more haphazardly matted in the arrangements of its fibers, giving it less elasticity than the original tissue. This means that the tissue on the edges of the scar is more prone to repeated injury if we overstrain again. Imagine a piece of fabric that has been torn and repaired by reinforcing it with a thicker substance than its original, like wax or some other adhesive substance. The actual repair site will be strong, but the edges of the repair will tear when the fabric is strongly stretched again.

The same thing happens in the tissues of the body. Areas of scar tissue formation will be tougher and less flexible and can become more prone to nearby injury in the future. It is best to avoid injury in the first place (and therefore the formation of scar tissue) by warming up well and by working carefully in good alignment. If an injury has occurred, we can help guide the healing process to encourage the scar to allow the degree of movement that we want. If we don't move, the scar tissue will develop to perpetuate the immobilized condition, becoming more of a restrictive bandage around the injury. Adhesions form in the connective tissue, which can cause pain and immobility. If we do use the injured part of our body even minimally, the newly formed tissue fibers will support the movement that we want for yoga practice. Bodywork and acupuncture can also help to bring more pliability to the scar tissue and prevent adhesions.

Fascia: The Grand Organizing Tissue

The fascial network of the body pervades every part of us, from head to toes, from just under the skin right down to the deepest layers of the body. The texture of fascia can be thin or thick, gel-like or more solid, depending on its local function. It provides internal structure and support, force transmission, and a source of sensory feedback. It separates and wraps around every organ, bone, muscle and blood vessel.

Each individual muscle is composed of bundles of fibers, each separated by thin layers of fascia, called **myofascia**. In the lower legs, the ankle muscles are separated from each other and organized into compartments by layers of fascia, just as thin layers of fiber separate the sections of an orange. You can think of those layers of fiber as a net that both supports individual segments and also connects those segments to the greater whole. The fascial "web" is continuous throughout the body, a fact that can be overlooked when we separate structures such as muscles, bones and organs in order to identify and study them. When we understand the all-pervasiveness of fascia, we see that moving one joint or even one part of the body never happens in isolation. Every movement pulls on the fascial web that connects above, below, around and across the body in many different patterns. Anatomist and bodywork trainer Thomas Myers maps out 12 specific myofascial meridians that transmit movement and strain throughout the body. His book *Anatomy Trains* is an excellent resource for study. Other fascial researchers have noted different patterns of fascial mapping. Another good source is *Fascia, the Endless Web: Fascial Anatomy and Physical Reality*, by R Louis Schultz and Rosemary Feitis. (See the Resources section for more information on these and other books on fascia.)

The sensations we feel during movement and exercise often come from the fascia, which has a more extensive sensory nerve supply than muscle tissue. In each chapter I will point out some ways that you can feel fascial connections in asana. Here's an example.

Try this now.
1. Place your legs in the wide stance for *Parshvakonasana* (Side Angle Pose).
2. Turn your right foot out at 90 degrees. Bend that knee and lean to the side. Notice that the stretch in your inner thighs may be the most evident sensation at first.
3. Now stretch your upper arm overhead alongside your ear. You would expect a shoulder stretch to come into the picture here, but due to the myofascial sheath that runs down the side of the body, when the arm goes overhead there is also a connected pull that occurs all the way down through the left ribs, hip and into the ankle and foot. It's not just the muscles and skin that are being stretched; it is also the myofascial line that surrounds and connects each individual muscle that is being highlighted and stretched.

Another example occurs in *Uttanasana* (Standing Forward Bend), a pose that stretches the entire myofascial sheath on the back of the body. Restrictions in that sheath anywhere along the line—from the back of the neck, through the spine, hips, legs and even the soles of the feet—may restrict our ability to bend forward with ease.

Try this now.

1. To perform Uttanasana, stand with your feet hip-width apart and parallel, and bow forward to touch the floor. If you are stiff, bend your knees slightly to avoid excessively rounding your lower back and to help your pelvis to tilt forward. Take note of the level of freedom or restriction you feel, and in which parts of your back body.

2. Stand up and apply pressure to the bottom of one foot by rolling it over a small rubber ball for a minute or more. This will evoke a release of the myofascia on the sole of your foot that will affect the entire back fascial sheath of the body, bringing you into a deeper forward bend on that side.

3. Test it out, and then repeat on the other side to balance the two sides.

When we stretch for more than a brief moment, our myofascia adapts to this new longer length and retains it, rather than recoiling. It is a moldable substance like plastic (think Silly Putty clay) and will hold its shape somewhat, but will tear if stretched too fast. It also becomes more pliable with heat. This molding effect can be best achieved through steady sustained stretching with the body warm. Bodywork can also mechanically stretch the myofascia. The details of all of these properties of fascia are still unfolding in current research.

Because fascia constitutes 30 percent of a muscle's bulk, the consistency of our fascia can be a significant factor in our overall flexibility. There are many different types of collagen with varying properties and degrees of flexibility. We are each born with a certain blend of these types of collagen. Even though our alignment and movements do make a huge difference to our flexibility in yoga, our heredity (and probably nutrition as well) will affect how easily we can touch our toes or wrap and fold ourselves into a wide range of yoga poses. Besides heredity and activity level, age is also a factor; our collagen stiffens as we age.

Although we cannot contract our fascia consciously like we can contract muscles, recent research has found that smooth muscle cells within the myofascia respond to surrounding stress by contracting. The myofascia can become chronically contracted and toughened in response to a misalignment of the skeletal structure. The body automatically braces to try to support itself, and the fascial tissue tightens in response. For instance, if you hold your hips to the right side for a prolonged period of time, the fascia and muscles on that side will become chronically thicker and tighter than the left side in the attempt to support the weight of your pelvis, which is off-center. Even though the muscles are in a stretched position, they remain in a state of chronic contraction, which anatomist Thomas Myers calls "locked long" (known in physiotherapy as "eccentrically loaded'). Conversely, the fascia and muscles on the other side will be "locked short" (or "concentrically loaded") and become weakened (*Anatomy Trains*, p. 301). In this situation, the resulting discomfort will probably be felt in the long side, but without opening the short side, we won't find balance. Stretching the aching long side will only increase the problem.

Ideally, fascia is resilient, meaning that it can respond to different types of demand, stretching and supporting as needed. It provides dynamic support and force transmission when we are moving, so it needs movement to keep it healthy. We can maintain its resiliency (its ability to recover quickly from any strain) by doing a variety of exercises. Fascia is toned by springy movements and stretched by holding a stretch position for at least 30 to 90 seconds. For a yoga practice, this means that a continuously moving vinyasa practice plus a series of poses held longer will give the fascia the variety of stimulus that it needs. Actively loaded stretches train the fascial layers best, in comparison to passive stretch or resistance training. An actively loaded stretch is one

in which the muscle being stretched is also contracting. This kind of stretch places a beneficial demand on the various types of fascia inside and around the muscle.

Being out of alignment over long periods of time can cause the fascia to become set in patterns that restrict our freedom. Thus, a frequent return to our own best possible alignment in our daily lives and in asana can help to maximize the resiliency and pliability of the fascia. It's not that we want to arrive at a fixed position that is "correct," but that we move in and out of a home-base position that is functionally balanced and free for our particular structure. The adventure of yoga is that we are constantly finding and redefining this goal as we practice throughout our lives.

Yogis have postulated that the fascia is the medium through which our *prana* (life force) flows. When the fascia is energetically balanced (not too tight or too loose, too long or too short) the pranic flow is stimulated, bringing great health to all cells of the body.

Because of the net of fascia pervading the body, we can see that the body structure is not just dependent on the shape and arrangement of bones. It is a dynamic structure in which the bones float in a continuous, supportive and mobile web of soft tissue. Because that web provides both stretchability (i.e., it is tensile) and integrity, Buckminster Fuller coined a term for it: **tensegrity**. In a tensegrity structure, none of the solid elements actually touch each other, but they are separated and supported by the softer tensile elements. The term "biotensegrity" is used to specify the tensegrity structure of the human body.

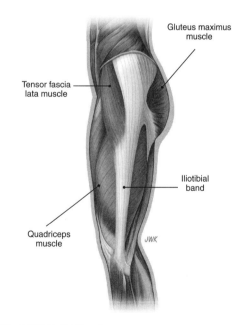

Figure 1.3a *Iliotibial band*

Gluteus maximus muscle

Tensor fascia lata muscle

Iliotibial band

Quadriceps muscle

JWK

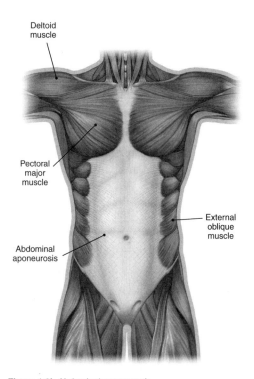

Figure 1.3b *Abdominal aponeurosis*

One band of fascia worthy of special note for yogis is the **iliotibial band** (see Figure 1.3a). This powerful support runs from the outer hip to the outer edge of the shin, crossing both the hip and knee joints. Two hip muscles attach to it superiorly, the gluteus maximus and the tensor fascia lata, tightening the fascia by pulling it from above. Its inferior (lower) attachment is just below the knee on the lateral (outer) side. The iliotibial band functions to help spread the load of work over the large thigh muscles and to stabilize us as upright two-legged beings. It reduces side-to-side wobbling in our hips when we walk or run, especially with the quick directional changes that happen frequently in sports and dance. When it becomes overly short, the iliotibial band

can cause movement restrictions in the hips, lower back or knees, often without localized pain but with cascading effects in these other joints. We stretch the iliotibial band in many standing poses, especially Utthita Trikonasana and hip openers such as *Eka Pada Rajakapotasana* (Pigeon Pose) preparation or *Agni Stambhasana* (Fire Log Pose).

Try this now.

1. With your hands, feel the texture of the fascia at the outer side of your thighs. Is it different from the texture of the quadriceps muscles at the front of your thighs or the hamstring muscles at the back?
2. Perform Utthita Trikonasana and notice the stretch of the iliotibial band on your back leg. Notice how you can

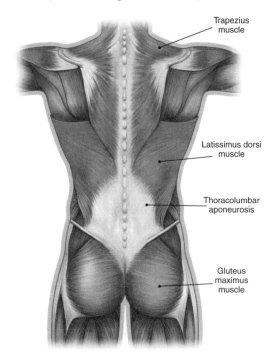

Figure 1.3c *Thoracolumbar aponeurosis*

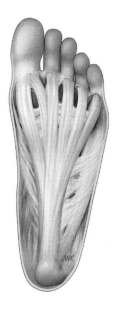

Figure 1.3d Plantar fascia

increase that stretch by stretching your upper arm horizontally over your ear and isometrically widening your back leg to the side as much as possible. This pulls on the continuous line of fascia down the side of your body.

Several other fascial tissues are worthy of note for yogis. The **abdominal aponeurosis** (and its central line at the front of the torso, called the **linea alba**) extends from the lower ribs to the pubic bone, and serves to protect the soft organs and provide attachments for the abdominal muscles (see Figure 1.3b). The **thoracolumbar aponeurosis** (serving as a tendon for large back muscles) is located at the back of the waist, and it serves to stabilize the lower trunk (see Figure 1.3c).

The **plantar fascia** spans the sole of the foot, connecting the heel to the toes and creating a bowstring that helps to support the longitudinal arch of the foot (see Figure 1.3d).

Proprioception

Often referred to as our sixth sense, our proprioception brings us information about the position of the body in space, or where each limb is in relation to the rest of the body. Along with our senses of sight, hearing, touch, taste and smell, this "sense" tells us about our spatial presence and our movements. It allows us to refine our postures and find our best alignment biomechanically. Our sense of proprioception tells us whether our arms are level in Virabhadrasana II, whether a knee is bent or straight in Utthita Trikonasana, or how much speed and force we will need to jump from Adho Mukha Shvanasana to Uttanasana. It also can bring us the delight of movement and physical expression in our practice. It gives us a vast array of signals every second of our lives, reporting in on how the body is shaped, whether we are still or moving, how fast and how intensely we are moving, and how to coordinate our movements and protect the body tissues. We have sensors in the smallest muscles, such as the ones that move our eyeballs, and in the largest ones, such as the thigh and hip muscles. As we practice yoga, we become more attuned to these proprioceptive messages, and therefore better able to use them effectively. This helps us to become more refined and sophisticated in our expression in the asana. This grand exchange of information takes place (for the most part) below the level of conscious thought.

As part of our proprioceptive capacity, we have sensors called **mechanoreceptors** within the joints and **reflexes** that coordinate the intricate balance of our muscle actions every moment of the day.

The Mechanoreceptors

Four types of receptors sense the mechanical functioning of the joints. These are located inside all synovial capsules in joints throughout the body. Types 1 and 2 tell us about angles, velocity and pressure within the joints. Type 3 warns about the limitations of range of movement in any joint, and Type 4 are the pain receptors, called nociceptors. Researchers postulate that people with hypermobility syndrome have less active nociceptors, allowing them to go too deeply into a stretch.

Reciprocal Inhibition

As mentioned earlier, most muscles operate in pairs as agonist and antagonist (muscles with opposite actions). The actions of the flexors are balanced by the action of the extensors, abductors are balanced by the adductors, and so on. This balancing and coordination occurs due to a reflex called **reciprocal inhibition**. Our nervous system is constantly balancing the use of each muscle in pairs of opposites to allow us to move in a coordinated and graceful way. When one muscle of a pair contracts (especially if the contraction is fast and strong), its antagonist automatically gets a reflex message to release,

allowing the agonist's movement to occur efficiently.

For instance, if we need to quickly contract the triceps to catch ourselves when jumping into *Chaturanga Dandasana* (Four-Limbed Staff Pose), the biceps will release, since this is a distinct agonist-antagonist pair of muscles. The nervous system inhibits the biceps when the triceps are active in order to increase the efficiency of the triceps. However, we can consciously override this reflex by contracting both agonist and antagonist together when we need extra joint stability. This is called **co-contraction**, and we use it frequently in yoga, though rarely by that name. For instance, in a seated forward-bending pose such as *Paschimottanasana* (Seated Forward Bend), contraction in the quadriceps helps the hamstrings to release, but we also simultaneously fire the hamstrings, which prevents overstretching and possible injury. In this way, the muscles cooperate without any one group overworking or overstretching. This kind of balanced use of muscles will support a healthy circulatory flow through the muscles and joints and a healthy range of motion. It also aids the fascia in remaining resilient and strong.

The Stretch Sensors

Within each muscle are specialized muscle fibers called **muscle spindles** that immediately respond to the degree of stretch and prevent a muscle from stretching too far or too fast. The fibers that sense stretch within the muscle (called **intrafusal** fibers) wrap around the muscle fibers like a spring. When they are stretched along with the muscle, they signal the muscle to contract at a level equal to the stimulus. A well-known example of this response is the "knee-jerk" test commonly performed by doctors: when a fast percussive pressure is applied to the tendon of the quadriceps tendon just below the knee, the pressure on the tendon pulls on the quadriceps muscle. The muscle spindle reports the stretch to the nervous system, which sends a reflex command to the muscle to contract, partially straightening the knee. We don't have to monitor this consciously; in fact, our brain is not even involved in creating the action. The message goes straight from the stimulus to the spinal cord and then immediately back to the muscle where a fast response is needed. Because of this reflex, "bouncing" in a stretch is counterproductive: the muscle you intend to stretch will respond to the speed of the stretch by contracting. When stretches are done too fast in this way, there is a likelihood of increased stiffness the next day.

The reaction of the intrafusal fibers is quick and strong, but its influence fades if the stretch continues at a steady rate. Moving into a stretch slowly and carefully avoids the activation of this reflex.

The Golgi Tendon Organs

The **Golgi tendon organs** were discovered by the scientist Camillo Golgi (1843–1926). Golgi tendon organs are sensors within the tendons that register the degree of tension in a muscle and signal the muscle to release in order to prevent tearing the tendon away from the bone. They maintain their influence over the muscle over a longer time than the muscle spindle. This characteristic of the Golgi tendon organs works to our advantage in yoga poses that we hold for at least 30 seconds. If we move into a pose slowly, the muscle spindles will be less likely to fire, and if we hold a pose longer, the Golgi tendon organs will be more likely to signal a muscular release. When the stimulus is gradual rather than sudden, the sensors recalibrate their reactions to the new length of the muscle, and our stretching is productive and satisfying.

Proprioceptive Neuromuscular Facilitation

Proprioceptive neuromuscular facilitation is a common stretching technique in the fitness world that takes advantage of the reflexes described above. In this method we alternate between contraction and stretch, using the built-in sensors to maximize the muscle's ability to stretch safely. An example will illustrate how it works.

Try this now.

Have a friend help you with this process, which involves working against resistance.

1. Lie on your back and lift one leg up perpendicular to the floor (Supta Padangushtasana).
2. Have your friend place their hand on the back of your heel where the Achilles tendon attaches.
3. Have your friend push on your heel to move your leg to the place that gives you a bit less than your maximum

hamstring stretch. Use your quadriceps to straighten the knee fully. This will engage the reflex of reciprocal inhibition and encourage an initial release of the hamstrings.

4. Staying at that angle, press your foot strongly into your friend's hand to about 80 percent of your maximum ability. This action contracts your hamstrings and therefore relaxes the stretch sensors in the muscle spindles. Hold this for about 10 seconds. The muscle spindles will reset to this new level of stretch. During this time the Golgi tendon organs will receive the stimulus of the contraction and signal the muscle to release more.

5. Next, release your pushing action against the resistance to a level about 20 percent of your maximum, and have your friend slowly move your leg into a position of deeper stretch. Keep the hamstrings slightly toned as they stretch. Moving too fast at this point will elicit the intrafusal fibers of the muscle spindles to tell the muscle to contract, so it is important to move slowly into the stretch. Reengage the quadriceps also, to bring back the reflex effect of reciprocal inhibition of the hamstrings.

6. Continue this alternation of contraction and release for a few cycles, and observe your range of motion increasing!

There are many variations of this type of stretching technique, and some researchers prefer the term "functional neuromuscular conditioning." For our purposes in yoga, we can be confident that stretching with muscular engagement around the joints and stretching slowly is not only safer, but also more effective in the long run.

In this chapter, I have outlined the basic anatomical information that you can apply to your study of the body. For example, you can picture the synovial capsule and ligaments that support each joint, and how the movements and shapes of yoga might affect those structures. You can experience the fascial net that both connects and separates your muscles and organs from each other as it responds to the pulls of a yoga pose. You can practice using pairs of muscles as agonists and antagonists, and observe the difference in feeling between a concentric contraction and an isometric contraction or between a faster stretch and a slower stretch. You can look up specific muscles for further study with the ability to understand the words used to describe the muscle's location and action. With these tools and preparation, you're ready for the next step: looking at each area of the body in depth.

Study Questions

1. Name the three spatial planes and indicate them with movements.

2. Define flexion, extension, abduction and adduction.

3. What are the three types of muscle tissue?

4. What are some types of connective tissue?

5. What is the difference between concentric and eccentric contraction? Give examples of each.

6. Name an agonist-antagonist pair of muscles and a yoga pose in which this pair is active.

7. What is a ligament? A tendon? An aponeurosis?

8. Where is fascia in the body? Describe some characteristics of fascia.

9. What is tensegrity? Give a yoga example of it.

10. What is reciprocal inhibition? How do we use it to stretch effectively in yoga?

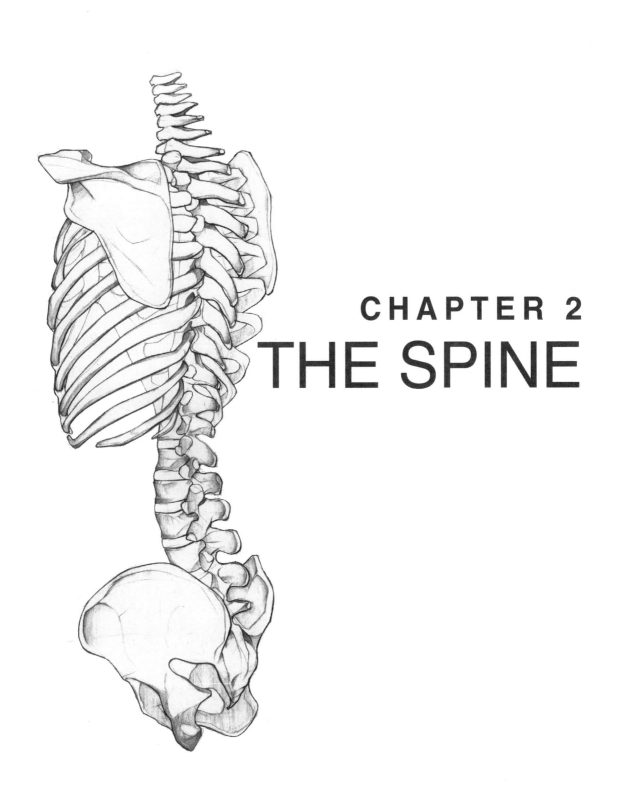

CHAPTER 2
THE SPINE

The spine is our central core, in both the biomechanical and spiritual aspects of who we are. Some say that the overall health of a person can be directly correlated to the health of the spine. As anyone with back pain can attest, we rely on its strength and movement in every activity of our day, and in resting as well.

In the Tantric view of the body, there are channels of energy throughout the body called *nadis*. The central one, the sushumna nadi, is located near the spine. It is through this channel that spiritual transformation takes place, making it essential to our path of hatha yoga. A healthy spine allows for a strong movement of prana through the subtle channels.

From the biomechanical viewpoint, the spine provides the support for our upright posture. In addition to supporting the weight of the entire upper body and transferring it to the legs, the spine provides many movement possibilities, due to its structure as a linked column of small bones and joints. The bones of the spine also protect the spinal cord, which contains the nerves that connect the brain to the rest of the body. It protects and carries the organs in our upright posture. Because of these three roles—weight bearing, movement and protection—the health of the body as a whole depends on the proper alignment and use of the spine and the muscles that move it.

In some sources the pelvis is considered to be part of the spine. The pelvis functions as the connecting link between the legs and the spine, and as such can be included in the study of either area. Here we will consider

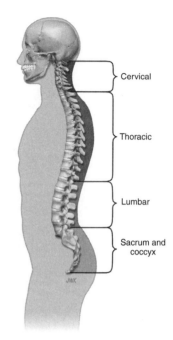

Figure 2.1 *Spine segments*

the spine as separate from the pelvis, since the pelvis is covered in Chapter Four. Neck muscles are covered in Chapter Seven.

The Bones and Discs of the Spine

The spine consists of a series of 24 vertebrae, each with several places of intersection with the adjoining ones. The spine is divided into three sections (see Figure 2.1): there are seven **cervical vertebrae**, 12 **thoracic vertebrae** and five **lumbar vertebrae** (see Figures 2.2a and 2.2b). The vertebrae are arranged like a stack of rings, the center of which is the housing for the spinal cord. Each vertebra has two main parts: the body, which is shaped like a lima bean and located toward the front, and the vertebral arch, the ring-shaped part at the back of the vertebra

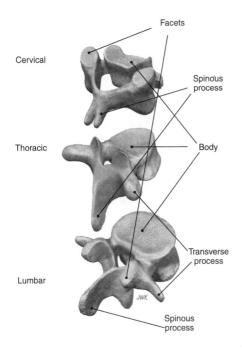

Figure 2.2a *Cervical, thoracic and lumbar vertebrae*

spinal cord is the bundle of nerves carrying impulses between the brain and the rest of the body. It is protected by three spoke-like appendages around the edges of the ring of the vertebra, which are features of each vertebra, but differing in shape in the different segments of the spine. There is one on each side, which are called **transverse processes**, and one at the back, called the **spinous process**. The spinous process is what you can feel under the skin as you touch someone's back. There is a small arch-shaped space at each side of each vertebra to allow for the spinal nerves to come out of the vertebral canal and go to the rest of the body (see Figure 2.4).

The discs are made of a thick outer layer called the **annulus** and a softer more liquid center called the **nucleus pulposus**, and they are affected by movement of the spine. Like the way a beanbag chair changes

that has spokes protruding from it. Between each of the vertebral bodies is an **intervertebral disc** providing spacing and cushioning. Each vertebra also touches its neighbors above and below via four **facet joints**. There are two facet surfaces reaching up (one on each side) and two facing downward (one on each side).

The top two vertebrae, the **atlas** and the **axis**, have a different structure from the rest of the vertebrae in order to support the head and provide maximum rotation. The atlas is like a ring, and the axis has a peg-like shape called the **dens** that fits inside the ring, a fit that allows ample rotation.

The **vertebral canal** or **foramen** is the hollow center of the stack of rings that forms a protective housing for the spinal cord. The

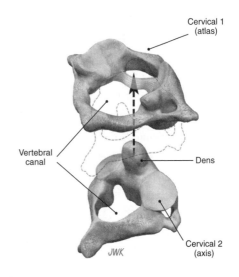

Figure 2.2b *Cervical vertebrae 1 and 2*

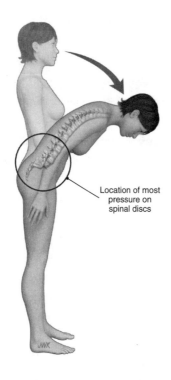

Figure 2.3a *Figure bending forward*

shape according to pressure from someone sitting in it, our discs adapt to pressure in the spine. When we forward bend, the disc pushes to the back, and when we backbend, it moves toward the front (see Figure 2.3b). Poor movement patterns and excessive forward-bending posture over a long period of time can cause the discs to push backward into the spinal canal. If the disc protrudes into the spinal canal, this is called a **bulging** or **protruding disc**. If the nucleus leaks out, it is called a **herniated or prolapsed disc** (see Figures 2.3b and 2.3c).

Aging causes shrinking and compression of the discs. If the disc shrinks, it will provide less spacing between the vertebrae, which will endanger the nerves as they exit from between

each vertebra. With less space between vertebrae, the movement range of the spine is decreased. Arthritis forms at the facet joints, which become compressed without the spacing provided by healthy discs. That wear and tear causes degenerative changes in the bones, resulting in arthritis (see Figure 2.4).

Discs are referred to by the numbers of their surrounding vertebrae and the first letter of the section of the spine, as in T12-L1 between the last thoracic and the first lumbar vertebrae, or L4-L5 between the fourth and fifth lumbar vertebrae. The lowest disc is a common problem area; it is L5-S1, the disc below the lowest lumbar vertebra and the sacrum. Its vulnerability comes from its position between the two large halves of the body: torso and legs. When we bend forward (especially with straight legs as in Fig 2.3a), the mechanical pressure on that segment of the spine may be enough to endanger the disc.

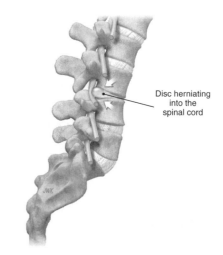

Disc herniating into the spinal cord

Figure 2.3b *Disc herniation lateral view*

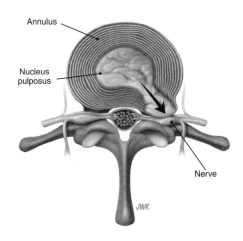

Figure 2.3c *Disc herniation superior view*

The Overall Shape and Movement Range of the Spine

The spine has natural curves in the sagittal plane, which add to the spine's resiliency. If the spine were straight, each step we take would jar our whole structure, causing an impact to the brain. The exact shapes of the curves vary with individuals, but in general the lumbar spine is concave as viewed from the back, the thoracic spine is convex and the cervical spine is concave (see Figure 2.1). The lumbar and cervical concave curves are called **lordosis**, both in normal range and also if the curve is excessive. The convexity of the thoracic spine is called **kyphosis**, both in its normal range and in excess. Any lateral curvature in the frontal plane is called **scoliosis**; mild scoliosis is quite common. Scoliosis can occur in small segments (one to three vertebrae) or larger segments (four or more vertebrae). The actual configuration is unique to each person with scoliosis and can be simple (one curve) or complex (several curves).

There is a difference in mobility in the different sections of the spine, based on the following factors: the shape and size of the vertebrae, the thickness of the discs, the attachments of the ribs to the thoracic section and the angle of the facet joint surfaces between the vertebrae. The cervical spine is well suited for flexion, extension and rotation but not as much for lateral flexion because of the shape of the transverse processes. The thoracic spine is well suited for flexion and some lateral flexion but not as much for rotation or extension due to constriction from the ribs. The lumbar spine is well suited for lateral flexion, flexion and extension, but it has very little rotation due to the orientation of the facet joints.

When sitting, we often lose the lordotic shape of the lumbar spine if it collapses and rounds. This is usually due to shortness in the posterior hip muscles (hamstrings and gluteus maximus) that does not allow

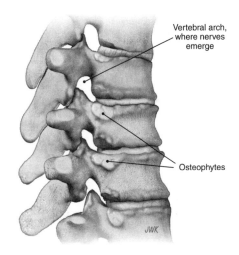

Figure 2.4 *Spinal arthritis*

sufficient hip flexion to maintain a neutral alignment of the pelvis. This is why it is so important to stretch the hamstrings for health of the lumbar spine. That last disc, L5-S1, receives too much pressure when the hamstrings are tight.

When we look at our own or someone else's spine, we can see what type of curves are there and attempt to be realistic about the types of movements that are possible. Someone with a flat lumbar spine will have more challenge in backbends, whereas someone with a more lordotic spine may have more challenge with forward bends. In general, we aim to maintain "normal" curves, then lengthen to create good support in the front and back of the spine. It's helpful to develop cues for yourself to help maintain the proper curves. For example, if you tend to have a flattened lumbar spine with very little curve, one useful cue is to take your upper thighs back. The femur bones serve as a lever to tilt the pelvis (more about this in Chapter Four). In contrast, if you have an excessive lumbar curve, you can try various cues: take the sides of the waistline back, firm and lift the lower abdominals and the pelvic floor, or lengthen the sacrum and tailbone downward.

Try this now.

With a partner, do the following:

1. Observe the cervical, thoracic and lumbar spinal curves in standing and sitting by touching the spinous processes.
2. Find the following landmarks: C7 at the base of the neck, T7 level with the bottom of the scapula, T12 level with the bottom of the ribs and L4 at the pelvic rim.
3. Observe the range of motion in each segment of the spine. To observe rotation in the lumbar spine, touch L1 and L4, then have the person do a seated twist. Observe whether your two fingers are still in line vertically or not.
4. Observe and touch the spine in Uttanasana to see if any segments or sections are deviated to the side in scoliosis.

The Ligaments of the Spine

There are three strong ligaments running the full length of the spine that protect the spine from excessive flexion (forward bending) and extension (backbending) (see Figure 2.5). One runs along the front of the vertebral bodies to prevent excessive extension, and two lie along the back (one inside the canal and one between the spinous processes) to prevent excessive flexion. There are other smaller ligaments as well, spanning only the space between two vertebrae.

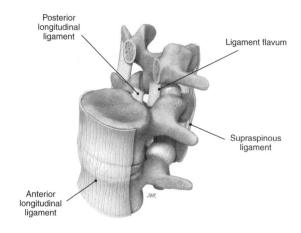

Figure 2.5 Spinal ligaments

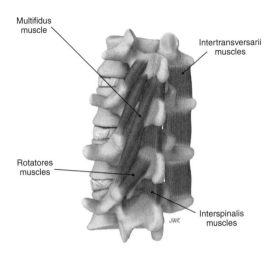

Figure 2.6 *Transversospinalis muscles*

The Muscles of the Spine

Those new to anatomy can get an overall understanding by visualizing the layers and seeing which muscles are small and which are large, with particular attention to groups two, three and four. Save the subcategories of each group for further study; just look at the big picture. We'll start with the deepest layers, then the intermediate layer, then the superficial layer.

Group One: Deep and Small Muscles

There are many small muscles that span two to six vertebrae. As a group they are called the **transversospinalis** (see Figure 2.6). Their actions are rotation, side bending and extension. The individual muscles are interspinales, intertransversarii, multifidus, rotatores and semispinalis. Though they are small, they function as our essential core support along with the abdominal muscles in front.

Group Two: Deep and Large Muscles

The **iliopsoas** originates at the sides of the lumbar vertebrae and runs down along the entire lumbar spine, through the pelvic bowl and across the hip joint to attach to the top of the inner femur (see Figure 2.7). It is made up of two muscles: the psoas major and the iliacus muscle. Contraction of the iliopsoas muscle, which is primarily a hip flexor, can cause flexion or extension of the lumbar spine, depending on which part of the muscle is more active. Contraction of the top part of the psoas results in spinal flexion, whereas contraction of the bottom part of the muscle results in spinal extension.

Try this now.

Because the iliopsoas is such a deep, large and uniquely shaped muscle, you need a sequence of four actions to stretch it effectively. Try this facing a wall, standing with your right leg forward and your left leg back, hands touching the wall for balance.

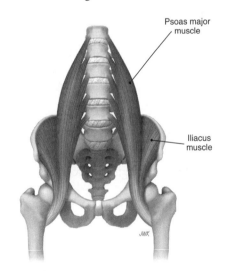

Figure 2.7 *Iliopsoas muscle*

1. Align the pelvis facing the wall and turn the back leg in slightly to align the iliopsoas muscle vertically.

2. Reach your left leg back to initiate the stretch in the lower part of the iliopsoas muscle. Your left heel can be off the floor.

3. Lengthen the back of the pelvis downward to stabilize the middle part of the iliopsoas muscle

4. Lift your front lumbar spine up to lengthen the top part of the iliopsoas muscle. You can arch your back and look up to engage the stretch of the upper iliopsoas.

5. All four of these actions are necessary in order to stretch the entire iliopsoas muscle.

The **quadratus lumborum** muscle originates on the iliac crest and inserts on rib 12 and to the sides of the lumbar vertebrae (see Figure 2.8). It is involved when we bend to the side (lateral flexion of the spine); one side will contract and the other side will stretch. It is also a strong support for the pelvis when standing on one leg, as in *Vrkshasana* (Tree Pose). You can feel it stretching in any side bend.

Try this now.

1. Do Utthita Trikonasana with your right foot pointing toward a wall and about 12 to 18 inches away from it. You can take your right arm to the floor or a block, or reach it to the wall.

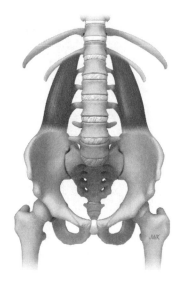

Figure 2.8 Quadratus lumborum muscle

2. Once you are in the pose, stretch your left arm up and over to the wall, increasing the stretch in the entire left side of your body. You will feel the quadratus lumborum stretching at the side of your waist.

Group Three: Intermediate Muscles
The **erector spinae (sacrospinalis)** is a group of muscles that fans outward and upward from its origin on the fascia of the lower back (see Figure 2.9). There are three divisions: one more lateral (iliocostalis), one a bit more medial (longissimus) and one near the spine (spinalis). They are further divided into sections according to which part of the spine they are located in: lumbar, thoracic, cervical or capitis (attaching to the head). They are active in any backbend and stretched in any forward bend.

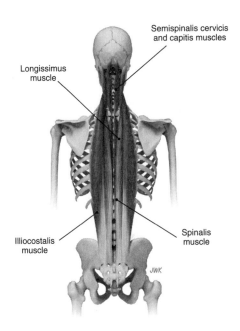

Figure 2.9 *Erector spinae muscles*

The **rhomboids** attach to the medial borders of the scapula and angle upward to attach to the thoracic vertebrae. They are actually shoulder muscles, but they help to extend the thoracic spine when they draw the scapula together. They are essential muscles for the support of the entire upper body. We stretch them in Garudasana (see Figure 7.5).

Try this now.

1. Either seated or standing, do a small backbend and feel the erector spinae muscles all the way down your spine.
2. Pull your scapulae together and feel the rhomboids contracting.

Group Four: Superficial Muscles

The **latissimus dorsi** is a very long and broad muscle that moves the arms back and moves the trunk into a backbend when the arms are weight bearing (see Figure 2.10). Its attachments are the thoracolumbar aponeurosis, the lumbar spine and pelvis, and the upper arm.

Try this now.

1. Stand tall and move your arm back as if putting on a coat. Notice the contraction all the way down into your lumbar spine; this is the latissimus dorsi stabilizing your back and bringing your arm back.
2. Now sit on the front edge of a chair or the floor, place your hands down behind you and lift your pelvis and spine up into a modified *Ushtrasana* (Camel Pose). This shows you the action of latissimus dorsi when your arms are weight bearing. We also use it to

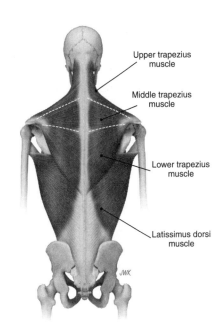

Figure 2.10 *Trapezius and latissimus dorsi muscles*

connect the arm into the shoulder, as in the upper arm of Parshvakonasana or both arms in Paschimottanasana.

The **trapezius**, also a shoulder muscle, is in three segments: upper, middle and lower (see Figure 2.10). It is shaped like a diamond, with its origin along the spine (and even onto the skull) from the top all the way down through the cervical and thoracic segments. Its upper segment extends the neck, as in *Bhujangasana* (Cobra Pose). Its middle segment pulls the scapula towards the midline (as in Sarvangasana), and its lower segment pulls the scapula down, which we do in many poses. All of these actions assist in extending and stabilizing the upper spine.

The Flexors of the Spine

We flex the spine (bending forward) by using the abdominal muscles, which are discussed in the next section. The only muscle that is directly attached to the vertebrae and could flex the spine is the upper psoas major muscle, part of the iliopsoas.

Try this now.

With a partner, observe the contraction of different muscle layers as your partner performs *Shalabhasana* (Locust Pose) with their arms to the side.

1. Feel the small muscles near the spine (transversospinalis) as they prepare to lift by firming those muscles into the core.
2. Feel the erector spinae and upper trapezius contract as they lift their head.
3. Feel the trapezius and latissimus dorsi contract as they lift their arms.
4. Feel the quadratus lumborum contract as they lift their legs.

The Big Picture

In a forward bend such as Paschimottanasana, you can feel the fascial connection from the erector spinae muscles down your entire back into the hamstrings, calves and feet. In the next exercise, you'll engage the whole fascial line first, then stretch it. Skip this exercise if you have a recent disc injury or other medical condition for which forward bending is contraindicated. Remember to keep breathing as you do this, and if the effort of the exercise blocks your breath, back off a bit.

1. Sit on one or two blankets if your hamstrings are tight. You can also place a rolled blanket under your knees if your hips are up on two blankets.
2. Place a bolster or folded blankets over your legs to rest your head on later.
3. Pull your upper thighs and buttocks back and apart with your hands, which will anteriorly tilt the pelvis. This will help free the pelvic movement.
4. Loop a belt around the soles of your feet and hold the ends of the belt.
5. Press your feet and legs down into the floor and lift your spine up (including your head and neck), engaging the entire back body and feeling the connections of each part.
6. Press your feet forward into the belt.
7. After toning the entire back body line in this way, retain some of that tone and begin to stretch forward. As you

fold forward, hinge at your hips as much as possible, pressing your sitting bones back as you tilt the top of your pelvis forward.

8. Notice the feeling of stretch as you pull your toes back with your hands or the belt, and as you bring your ribs forward toward your feet. You can adjust the position of your hands on the belt as needed or grasp your feet directly. Notice whether the sensation changes when you bow your head forward toward your legs. The chain of muscles and fascia includes the fascia that surrounds your skull, your spinal extensors, your gluteal muscles, your hamstrings, gastrocnemius, and foot and toe flexors. Each part of the inter-connected chain makes its contribution to the distribution of force and stretch. You might feel it much more in some areas because of your particular fascial patterns, but see if you can feel the entire line.

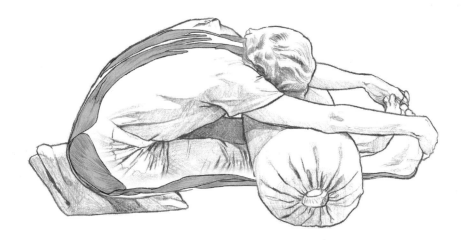

Study Questions

1. What three functions does the spine fulfill for us?

2. Name the three sections of the spine and the number of vertebrae in each. Which are most mobile? Why?

3. What part of the vertebrae can you touch on someone's back?

4. Describe the location of the spinal cord and how the nerves emerge from it.

5. How does movement affect the spinal discs? Why is it important to move the spine in all the directions it can move?

6. Define kyphosis, lordosis and scoliosis.

7. Name the group of deep and small back muscles.

8. Name the two deep and large back muscles.

9. Name the three-part intermediate layer back muscle that is our main back-bending muscle.

10. Name the two superficial muscles on the back.

11. Choose five yoga poses and analyze the spinal actions in each, naming as many of the muscles involved as you can. Include the fascial connections to other parts of the body as well.

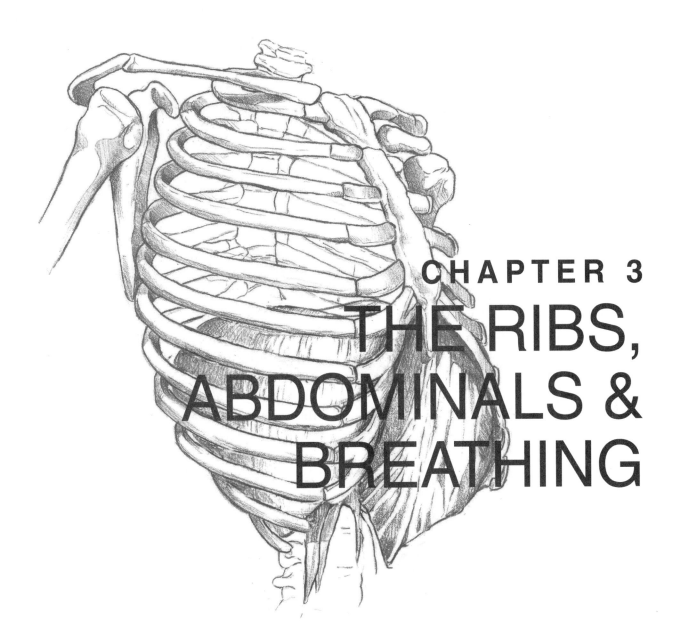

CHAPTER 3
THE RIBS, ABDOMINALS & BREATHING

One of yoga's greatest benefits is to help people to breathe more fully. By stretching all sides of the torso, the spine, ribs and lungs become more elastic, allowing the breath to expand. When the breath is smooth, steady and full, we nourish the body with oxygen, and we also calm the mind. Prana, the essence of the breath, moves freely through us, and our overall health improves. In this chapter we outline the main muscles of breathing, and we explore the relationship of the abdominal muscles to both posture and breathing. Throughout this study of the breath, remember that prana is our true source of vital energy and healing.

The Sternum, Ribs and Clavicles

The sternum and ribs enclose the thorax (chest), protecting the lungs and the heart (see Figure 3.1). The sternum is a long, flat bone with three parts: the manubrium at the top, the body in the middle and the xiphoid process at the lower end.

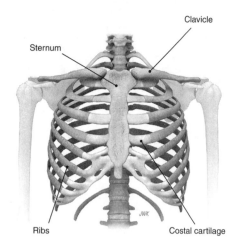

Figure 3.1 Sternum, ribs and clavicle

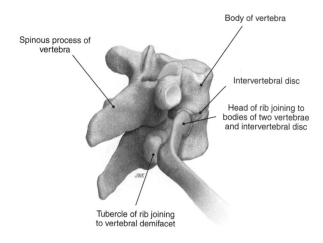

Figure 3.2 Rib attachment to vertebra

There are 12 ribs, which each attach in the back to the associated thoracic vertebra via three small joints on each rib (see Figure 3.2). In the front, the attachments of the ribs are as follows: The first seven ribs attach directly to the sternum, and these are called "true" ribs. The next three, ribs 8–10, attach to the costal cartilage and then to the sternum and are called "false" ribs. The last two, ribs 11 and 12, do not attach at all in the front, and they are called "floating" ribs.

Each section of the ribs has a characteristic direction of movement when we inhale. The top ribs expand upward, the middle ribs expand to the side, and the lower ribs expand downward and outward. This movement is often described as being similar to the way a bucket handle moves.

The ribs move up and down thanks to two layers of muscles between each rib, called the **intercostals**. The external intercostals expand the ribs for inhalation, and the internal intercostals contract the ribs for forced exhalation, sneezing, coughing, and so on.

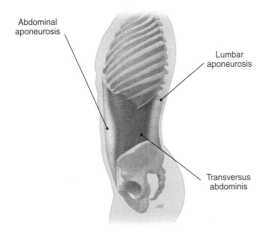

Figure 3.3a Transversus abdominis

The two clavicles (collar bones) span the top of the front chest, articulating with the sternum at the center and with the scapula on each side (see Figure 3.1). Their purpose is to connect the shoulder girdle to the central core of the body. They move with any arm movement.

In yoga we often use cues relating to these bones in order to lift the spine and stand tall. We say "Lift your sternum" or "Lengthen your side ribs" or "Lift and broaden your collar bones."

Try this now.

1. Take a series of deep breaths to feel the movement of your ribs, clavicles and sternum.
2. Touch someone else's ribs to feel the same movement.
3. Experiment with different instructional cues to help lift and broaden the front chest and spine in yoga poses.

The Abdominal Muscles

The transversus abdominis

There are four layers of abdominal muscles that function to support and compress the abdomen, flex the spine and twist the torso. The deepest is the **transversus abdominis**, which wraps like a belt around the waistline (see Figure 3.3a). It is really a "side" muscle, since it attaches to the broad abdominal fascia in front and to the broad lumbar fascia in back. In addition, it attaches to the lower ribs, the xiphoid process of the sternum and the top of the pelvis.

The internal and external obliques

The next layer superficial to the transversus abdominis is the **internal oblique**, whose fibers run obliquely upward and medially from the pelvic crest to the lower ribs (see Figure 3.3b). Superficial to that is the **external oblique**, whose fibers run along the opposite diagonal, downward and medially

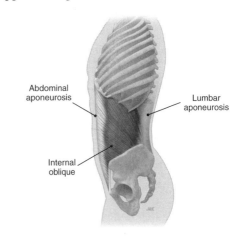

Figure 3.3b Internal oblique

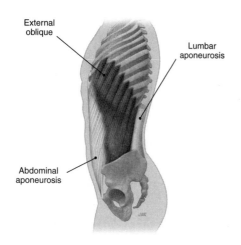

Figure 3.3c *External oblique*

toward the pubic bone (see Figure 3.3c). These two muscles help us to twist the torso. Make a mental note that any muscle whose fibers are oriented at a diagonal, wrapping around the body, is involved in twisting.

The rectus abdominis

The most superficial abdominal muscle is the **rectus abdominis** (see Figure 3.4). Its origin is the pubic bone and its insertion is on ribs 5–7. Contraction of this muscle flexes the spine. We can use it in sections, as when we contract only the lower or the upper segments of the muscle. The fascia surrounding the rectus abdominis is continuous with the fascia of the pelvic floor. Because of this, when we lift the pelvic floor, the lower fibers of the rectus abdominis will contract, which provides good support for the lumbar spine.

Significance of the Abdominals in Yoga

The abdominals are important for spinal support, but if over-exercised, they can cause shortening of the front body. This is especially common in people who spend much of their time sitting or standing with slumped posture, or those who practice multiple sit-ups or abdominal crunches. Shortness in the front body makes backbends more difficult because the ribs are pulled downward by the upper part of the rectus abdominis, restricting spinal extension. Short abdominals can also lead to neck alignment problems and breathing restrictions. It is important to stretch the abdominals with poses like Bhujangasana and Urdhva Dhanurasana to maintain length in the front torso. In all backbends, long abdominals will allow the entire spine to participate in the backbending action.

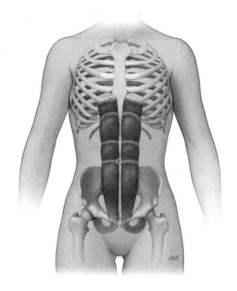

Figure 3.4 *Rectus abdominis*

We use the abdominals not only to flex the spine, but in twisting as well. The obliques assist the transversospinalis muscles to twist the spine, working on one side at a time. The abdominals are also key players in arm-balancing poses, holding the trunk steady as you balance over your hands.

Try this now.

1. Consciously contract each layer separately as much as you can.
2. To isolate the transversus, pull in your waistline.
3. To isolate both layers of the obliques, twist your torso. When you twist to the right, your left external oblique and your right internal oblique will be working.
4. Reverse this to the other side.
5. To isolate the rectus abdominis, pull your pubic bone up and your front ribs down. Notice how this shortens your front torso.

Prana

The breath is our most direct connection to the universal energy of prana that sustains us. The air we breathe becomes the vehicle for the prana, or vital force, and as such it feeds every cell of the body. Our responses to the environment around us, both physiologically and emotionally, are contained in the breath. The breath forms a concrete link between the physical body and the subtle body, giving us access to one from the other, allowing us to revitalize or calm ourselves as needed. Respiration is the only vital bodily function that is maintained automatically but can also be under our voluntary control, as in the practice of pranayama. Knowing how the breath works physiologically gives yoga practitioners and teachers the opportunity to observe and practice the poses in a way that optimizes the flow of prana.

The Muscles of Breathing

The **diaphragm**, our primary breathing muscle, is a double-dome-shaped muscle suspended across the middle of the trunk (see Figures 3.5 and 3.6). It forms the division between the thoracic cavity and the abdominal cavity. It is unlike any other muscle in that it attaches to its own central tendon at the top, rather than attaching to a bone at the top. The sides and lower part of the dome attach to three bony

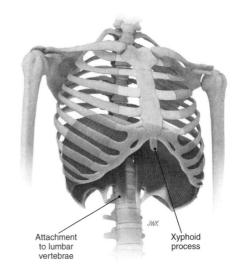

Attachment to lumbar vertebrae

JWK

Xyphoid process

Figure 3.5 Diaphragm oblique view

43

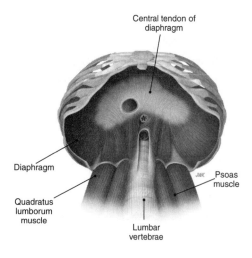

Figure 3.6 *Diaphragm inferior view*

connections on all sides of the torso: the xiphoid process of the sternum in front, the inside of the lower ribs around the sides and the sides of the first few lumbar vertebrae at the back. You could compare its shape to a double-domed parachute. When the diaphragm muscle contracts, it pulls downward. Because it is attached via soft tissue to the underside of the lungs, it expands the lungs as it pulls down, and air is pulled in. Then as the diaphragm relaxes, it moves back up again, and the air is pushed out by the natural elasticity of the lung tissue. Because its contraction pulls downward, it will tend to push the abdominal organs down, causing a swelling of the abdomen on inhalation.

Note: Some call this belly-expanding breath "diaphragmatic breathing" as opposed to "chest breathing," where we mostly depend on expansion of the ribs to fill the lungs. In fact, all breathing is diaphragmatic; the difference can be in the amount of movement we allow in each part of the chest.

Try this now.

1. Take a few breaths, experimenting with expansion in different parts of your ribs (lower, middle, upper, front and back). There is no one correct way to breathe: the ideal breath is one that responds appropriately to the demands of what we are doing.

2. Notice that you can allow your belly to expand as you inhale, or you can restrict it from expanding with your abdominal muscles. How does each way of breathing feel different?

The diaphragm is pierced by three openings to allow three important structures to pass through: the esophagus (carrying food to the stomach), the inferior vena cava

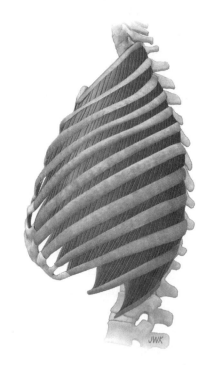

Figure 3.7a *External intercostals*

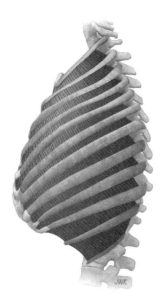

Figure 3.7b Internal intercostals

(a major vein carrying blood from the lower body to the heart) and the aorta (a major artery carrying blood from the heart to the lower body).

The Secondary Breathing Muscles

The intercostals

The **intercostals**, two layers of muscles located between each rib, are arranged at diagonals so that they can efficiently pull the ribs up and out like bucket handles. This action expands the chest cavity to make room for the air we breathe into the lungs. The two layers are the external intercostals and the internal intercostals (see Figures 3.7a and 3.7b).

The scalenes

The **scalenes** are three muscles at the sides of the neck that assist in forced inhalation by lifting the top two ribs (see Figure 3.8). To feel their action, touch the sides of your neck and take a quick and fast breath in, as if you are about to sneeze. You will feel the scalenes contract as they lift the top ribs to help fill the lungs. These muscles are also an important support for the neck and head, as in Utthita Trikonasana, when the head is held to the side. When going to the right in Utthita Trikonasana, the left scalenes will be active. When going to the left side in the pose, the right scalenes will be active.

Breathing and the Abdominals in Yoga

For many beginners, the breath is restricted by inflexibility of the ribs or by collapse of the thoracic spine. The good news is that all types of yoga poses can help bring strength and flexibility to these areas for better breathing.

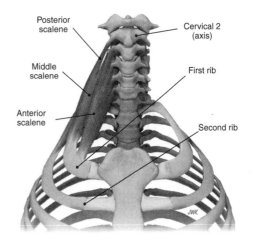

Figure 3.8 Three scalene muscles

45

Forward bends stretch the back of the ribs and lungs, backbends stretch the front and side bends stretch the side. Twists stretch the diaphragm and the intercostals.

When performing asana or any exercise, it is wise to use the abdominals for support of the lower back. However, when the abdominals work strongly, they prevent the abdominal cavity from changing shape in response to the downward movement of the diaphragm. In other words, it can be difficult to get a satisfying deep breath. For instance, in arm balances or other strenuous poses, we need to breathe more into the upper lungs and less into the lower lungs. Because the breath is less deep, it moves more quickly to bring in enough oxygen. We get "out of breath," and we instinctively breathe more deeply after coming out of the pose. Then the question to ask is: What happens when that strong abdominal support is no longer necessary? Can we return to a more relaxed breathing pattern?

If we develop a habit of always breathing "higher" in the rib cage, this can contribute to anxiety and reduced capacity for relaxation. However, with awareness we can vary the use of our abdominals as needed: For strenuous poses like arm balances, full contraction of the abdomen is useful to integrate the trunk of the body with the legs. For poses requiring moderate exertion, like standing poses, we can keep some tone in the lower abdomen to support the lumbar spine while still allowing the upper abdomen to remain soft, so that the lower ribs can move down to fill the lower lungs. Then during *Shavasana*

(Corpse Pose) we can allow the abdomen to soften completely and the breath to deepen more. This kind of refined use of the abdominals in breathing is a major benefit of asana and pranayama practice.

Other Physical Aspects of Breathing

Gas exchange takes place inside the lungs in small sac-like structures called **alveoli**, which look like bunches of grapes. Blood vessels surround these alveoli, and gas exchange occurs across the cell membranes that form the "skin" of each alveolus. If you spread out the membranes of all the alveoli of one person, the actual gas-exchange surface area, it would be about half the size of a tennis court.

We breathe approximately 23,000 times a day, 900 times in one hour, 15 to 20 times a minute.

The normal volume of air that goes in and out is called the **tidal volume**. We can increase that amount during inhalation, taking in an **inspiratory reserve volume**. Exhaling as much as possible shows us the **expiratory reserve volume**. **Vital capacity** is the sum of all three of these amounts. Yoga practice increases our vital capacity, enlivening all of our cells and the mind as well.

Inhalation is correlated with nervous system arousal, whereas exhalation is correlated with relaxation. A healthy heart rhythm demonstrates this moment-to-moment fluctuation, which is called **respiratory sinus arrhythmia**. Scientists now recognize that heart rate variability is an indicator of overall health, as described in Roger Lewin's book *Making Waves*.

Try this now.

1. Find the place on your forearm near your wrist on the thumb side where your pulse is evident.

2. Spend a few minutes breathing normally, and see if you can feel your pulse speed up slightly as you inhale and slow down slightly as you exhale.

The Big Picture

Connect the entire upper side body in *Ardha Chandrasana* (Half-Moon Pose). Proceed with care or skip this pose if you have significant balance problems or other contraindications for standing on one leg. Stay in touch with your breath as you explore the pose.

1. Standing with your back to a wall for stability, place your right foot parallel to the wall.

2. Bend your right knee and bring your right hand to the floor or a prop (a block or chair) about 12 to 18 inches away from your right toes. Lift and extend your left leg behind you along the wall, pointing the toes away from the wall. Your left hand can stretch up or rest on your side hip.

3. Notice your side neck muscles (scalenes) supporting the weight of your head. That support transfers to your intercostals and oblique abdominals, then into your hip muscles and fascia (gluteals, tensor fascia lata, iliotibial band) and into the peroneals at the side of your lower leg and foot.

4. Lift your head and left foot, toning the entire chain of muscles and fascia, then stretch it as you slightly lower your head and foot. Notice the connection from your left ear all the way to the left outer foot.

5. Explore how awareness of your breath can help you do this pose.

6. Repeat on the other side.

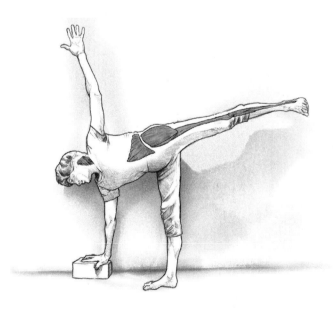

Study Questions

1. How many ribs do we have?

2. Where do the ribs attach?

3. Describe the movement of the ribs in breathing.

4. What two other bones does the clavicle connect to?

5. Name the muscles of respiration and describe their location.

6. Describe the action of the diaphragm in a normal breath.

7. What are the four layers of abdominal muscles?

8. Why is abdominal strength important in yoga, and how can it also be detrimental?

9. Pick a pose and discuss with a friend how the intercostal and abdominal muscles are used in the pose, and how they link up with other muscles through the fascial lines.

10. Describe some ways in which your breathing has improved from your yoga practice.

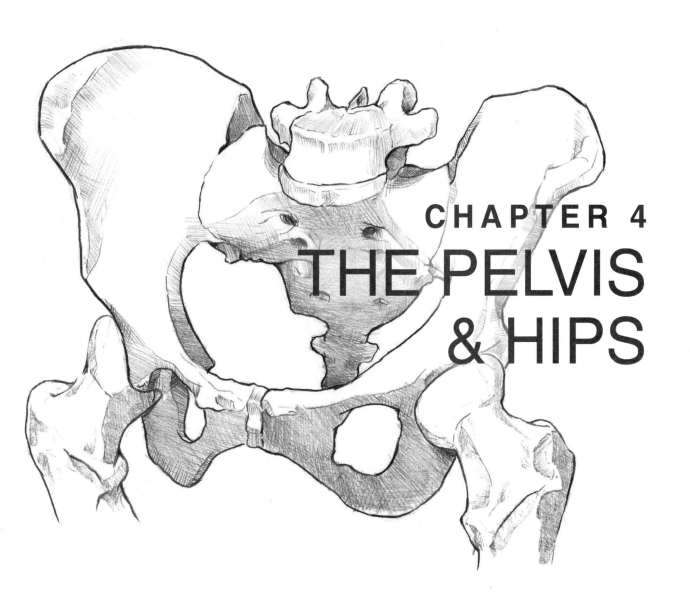

CHAPTER 4
THE PELVIS
& HIPS

To understand the biomechanics and beauty of our posture, balance, locomotion and virtually all essential human activities, we need to understand the pelvis. A complex structure with many moving parts, the pelvis is the central organizing structure from which everything else in the body can be seen to emerge. If we think of the body as a temple, the pelvis is its cornerstone, its core. Through the pelvis, the weight of the entire upper body is transferred to our two legs, so it functions as a biomechanical intersection. Any force created by walking, running or jumping is transmitted to the upper body through the pelvis. You can also think of it as a bowl or vessel that protects and cradles the digestive and reproductive organs, and in childbearing, the growing fetus. In fact, the word "pelvis" is from the Latin word for "basin." In that basin, new life is created.

In yoga subtle anatomy, the pelvis is the location of the *kanda*, or bulb. The kanda is the origin of the sushumna nadi and all the subtle energy channels through which prana flows.

The Bones of the Pelvis and Thigh

The adult pelvis is made up of five bones, some of which are fused together.

The ilia

The **ilia** (singular: **ilium**) are the two curved sides of the bowl. The top rim of each ilium is called the **iliac crest**. You can touch your iliac crest and follow the curve from the front to the back. In the front,

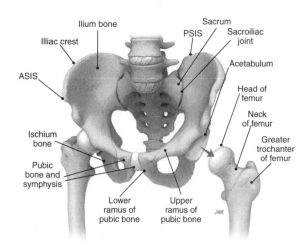

Figure 4.1 *Pelvis and femur*

the prominent corner is called the **anterior superior iliac** spine, or **ASIS**. At the back, there is another knob as the curvature of the top rim ends in the sacroiliac joint; this is called the **posterior superior iliac spine**, or **PSIS**. These are good landmarks to know.

The ischia

The **ischia** (singular: **ischium**) are the curved bones at the lower part of the pelvis. They are continuous with the ilia, meaning there is no joint between them, and anatomists have arbitrarily designated where the ilium ends and the ischium begins. The most important parts of the ischia are the **ischial tuberosities**, or the sitting bones. You can feel them by reaching under your pelvis while sitting.

The pubis

The **pubis** is the two-part bone at the front lower pelvis. You probably know it as the bony prominence you can feel at the front, but there's more to it. From front and center, the pubis continues back on the left and right sides to connect with the ilium above (the **upper ramus**) and below to the ischium (the **lower ramus**). These landmarks (the two rami) are important because they are the places of attachment for the adductor muscles.

The sacrum

The **sacrum**, or "sacred bone," is the blade-shaped bone that fits between the two ilia at the back and forms the base for the 24 spinal vertebrae. It is formed by five vertebrae that fuse together during the first two decades of life. The sacrum is also a double-layered pocket with a back and front side, somewhat like a pita bread. There is an opening at the top for the large bundle of nerves coming down from the spinal cord. Nerves exit from holes in the sacrum and from behind the sacrum to go down the legs.

The coccyx

The **coccyx**, or tailbone, is the small vestigial tail at the base of the sacrum, with three or four vertebral segments. Sizes and shapes of the tailbone vary greatly from one person to another.

The femur

The **femur** is the thigh bone, whose head inserts in the acetabulum to form the hip joint, or iliofemoral joint (see Figure 4.1). Though the femur is not a pelvic bone, I include it here because this chapter covers the hip joints as well as the pelvis. Note its

shape, like the number 7 (a somewhat horizontal portion, a corner, then a vertical portion). The head of the femur is connected to the neck, which ends in a large prominence at the corner called the **greater trochanter**, which you can feel on the side surface of your hip. Then the bone turns downward, angling in slightly to form the top part of the knee joint.

When you look at a picture of all these bones together, you may notice that the "bowl" of the pelvis is not solid on all sides, and it is more open at the front. There are open spaces and curved struts that allow for the pelvis to be light as well as strong. Notice in particular the **obturator foramen** (see Figure 4.2a), the rounded opening toward the lower part of the pelvis above the ischial tuberosities, which is an attachment site for some of the pelvic floor muscles. In general, the male pelvis is longer and narrower, and the female pelvis is wider to allow for childbearing.

The Joints of the Pelvis

The lumbosacral junction

Moving from top to bottom, the first joint of the pelvis is the **lumbosacral junction**. The fifth lumbar sits on top of the sacral promontory, a small platform. This is a site of frequent disc strain, when the upper body curves forward but the pelvis is stationary.

The sacroiliac joints

The sacroiliac joints are formed by the sides of the triangle-shaped sacrum fitting between

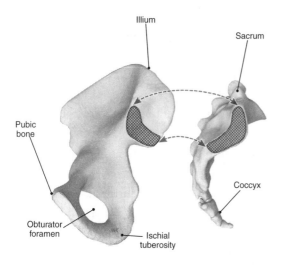

Figure 4.2a *Sacroiliac joint separated*

the joint surfaces of the two ilium bones, one on each side (see Figures 4.1, 4.2a and 4.2b). These joints are oriented obliquely (not straight either from side to side or front to back). The surface of the joint is irregular, and the two bones fit together like three-dimensional moonscape puzzle pieces, with hills and valleys nestled together.

The iliofemoral joint

The **iliofemoral joint** (hip joint) is a ball-and-socket joint formed by the **acetabulum** (the socket) and the head of the femur bone (the ball). The acetabulum (Latin for "little vinegar cup") is located at the front and side of the pelvis. The socket itself is formed by one-third ilium, one-third ischium and one-third pubis.

For stability and joint health, it is ideal to have the femur head fully and evenly placed in the acetabulum. If it is constantly pushed to one side or constantly turned forward or back, it can unevenly wear out the cartilage that lines the inside of the hip joint. For this reason, doing a complete variety of movements for this joint is essential to maintain its health. In other words, we need to do flexion, extension, abduction, adduction, external rotation and internal rotation. The alignment principles of yoga (see below) help us to position the femur in the center of the acetabulum as much as possible. When we turn the legs in, then move the femurs back and widen them, this complex but essential action places the femoral head back and out to the side in the hip socket. We balance that action with its opposite, drawing in from the sides of the hips and rotating the legs externally for stability. These opposite actions (performed together) will balance the femur in the acetabulum. We'll see later in this chapter which muscles perform each of those actions.

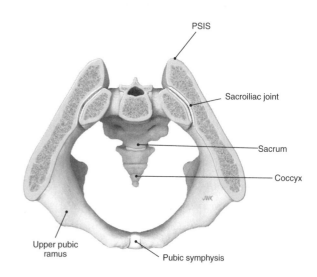

Figure 4.2b *Sacroiliac joint cross section (superior view)*

The pubic symphysis

The **pubic symphysis** is the joint between the two parts of the pubis; it is a semi-move-able joint that can expand for childbirth. This joint has an articular disc like those between the 24 spinal vertebrae.

The sacrococcygeal joint

The **sacrococcygeal joint** can move a bit. In some people, the segments of the coccyx also move independently, like the spinal vertebrae.

Try this now.

Touch as many of these bones, joints and landmarks as you can, naming each one.

The Ligaments of the Pelvis

All joints in the body are supported by ligaments that hold the bones in their relative positions. The lumbosacral junction, often called L5-S1 to denote the fifth lumbar

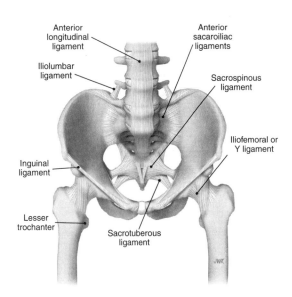

Figure 4.3b Anterior pelvic ligaments

vertebra sitting on the first sacral vertebra, has many small ligaments that secure the lowest lumbar vertebrae to the ilia and the sacrum, and another ligament that covers the fronts of the vertebrae. These ligaments run vertically, diagonally and horizontally. The sacroiliac joint has ligaments on both the anterior and posterior sides, forming a secure web for the bones (see Figures 4.3a and 4.3b).

The thin **inguinal ligament** (in the front) runs from the pubic bone up and laterally to the ASIS. The larger **sacrotuberous ligament** (in the back) runs from the sacrum to the ischial tuberosity, or sitting bone. The **sacrospinous ligament** (also in the back) runs from the sacrum to the ischial spine, a prominence that is above the ischial tuberosity.

The **iliofemoral ligament** encircles the hip joint. It is also called the **Y ligament**, since it looks like the letter Y from the front.

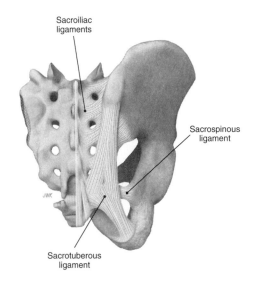

Figure 4.3a Posterior sacroiliac ligaments

Parts of this ligament arise from the ilium, ischium and pubis and wrap around the head of the femur, securing it in the socket yet allowing it a full range of motion.

All ligaments are affected by our movement and by our body chemistry. Stress and fatigue weaken the ligaments, and for women, the monthly hormonal shift can bring changes in ligament stability. In pregnancy, the hormone relaxin softens all the ligaments to make the pelvis ready for the growing fetus.

The Pelvic Tilt

Because the pelvis rests on two round surfaces (the femur heads), it can tilt in different directions, which is significant for our posture. Anterior tilt is defined as the movement forward at the top of the pelvis (the iliac crest; see Figure 4.4.a), and posterior tilt is defined as the reverse, in which the iliac crest moves back (see Figure 4.4b). Anterior tilt is also called nutation, and posterior tilt is called counter-nutation.

Try this now.

1. Try these two types of tilt in several different positions: standing, sitting, and on your hands and knees.
2. You will notice that anterior tilt also brings an arched shape to the lumbar spine, which is called lumbar extension or lordosis.
3. Posterior tilt conversely brings a flat or rounded shape to the lumbar spine, which is called lumbar flexion or kyphosis.
4. Can you find the place in the middle, as in the neutral tilt pictured in Figure 4.4c?

The optimal alignment of the pelvis is a neutral tilt, which maintains the normal slight lordotic curve of the lumbar spine. When we hold the pelvis in posterior tilt for long periods of time, such as slouching when we sit at a desk or in a car, this creates strain on the lumbar discs and all the lumbar soft tissue. Unfortunately, many chairs and car seats are built to accommodate the slouch, rather than helping us to sit tall. It is especially dangerous for the discs if you lift a heavy object while the lumbar spine is in flexion. Even though we need to use our abdominal muscles strongly to stabilize the spine while lifting, we also need to maintain the neutral spinal shape, using strength from all sides evenly. This protects the discs. One way to help adjust your seated posture and create the proper tilt of the pelvis is to manually pull your buttocks back and apart. This will allow for the normal arch of your lumbar spine and create good support for the entire upper body.

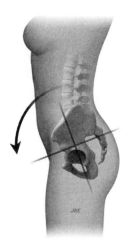

Figure 4.4a *Anterior tilt*

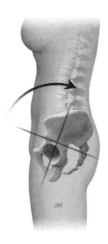

Figure 4.4b *Posterior tilt*

Try this now.

1. Experiment with your pelvic tilt in various different positions: lying supine, sitting, standing, on hands and knees, and leaning forward from standing.

2. Create a moderate lumbar arch by pulling your sitting bones and buttocks back and apart, then lift your abdominals without causing spinal flexion. This is the kind of support the spine needs when you are lifting heavy objects.

Sacroiliac Movement

In the section above we defined the movements that occur on both sides of the pelvis at once: anterior and posterior tilt of the whole pelvis. The sacroiliac joint also moves a small amount throughout our normal daily movements, either both sides at once or differently on the right and left sides. For instance, when you step forward with your right foot, your right ilium will tilt posteriorly to help that leg move forward as the back

of the pelvis lengthens. Conversely, the left ilium will tilt anteriorly to allow the left leg to go back. This movement is moderated in the sacroiliac joint.

Try this now.

1. Walk very slowly to feel the movement of your pelvis on each side.

2. Try a more extreme movement forward with your right leg, such as a marching step, a lunge pose in yoga, climbing up two or three stairs at once, or *Hanumanasana* (Leaping Monkey Pose). This movement (different on the two sides) will be greater in the sacroiliac joint. One side tilts forward, the other side tilts back, and a healthy sacroiliac joint will allow this.

The sacroiliac joint could be strained in twisting poses if we do not stabilize the pelvis strongly. The sacrum needs to stay centered between the two ilia, with the spinal twist

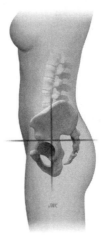

Figure 4.4c *Neutral tilt*

occurring above the pelvis, incrementally up the entire spine. With normal alignment, supportive action and ligament health, a good range of movement, including twists, can be accomplished. But if the joint is stuck, misaligned or unstable, a demand for movement may cause pain. Careful attention to stretching and strengthening the surrounding soft tissue evenly will help to prevent most sacroiliac dysfunction. As we discuss the muscles, we will note which ones are particularly involved in sacroiliac support. When misaligned, the sacroiliac joint may realign itself as we practice yoga, or we may need to seek help to resolve the problem.

The Muscles of the Pelvis

We will examine the muscles in seven groups: the hip flexors, the hip extensors, the hip adductors, the hip abductors, the hip medial rotators, the hip lateral rotators and the pelvic floor. Then we will note which muscles are most important for sacroiliac support and which muscles perform certain key actions in yoga. You will see that many of the hip muscles perform several different tasks, so they fit into more than one of these functional groups. In fact, most muscles of the body are multitaskers; this is what makes the study of human movement so fascinating! Muscles do not work in isolation; they work as teams, and their actions can vary according to which members of the teams are playing at any given time. If you are just beginning your study of anatomy, focus on the primary muscles listed below. Later, you can expand your viewpoint to include the assisting muscles, noting what nuances each one contributes to the action you are considering. Note that the muscles with a larger span of attachment tend to be efficient multitaskers. Watch especially for gluteus medius in this regard.

After reading about each group, try a pose that strengthens each muscle, and one that stretches each.

The Primary Hip Flexors
The iliopsoas

The **iliopsoas**, which you met in Chapter Three as a spinal muscle, is a large, deep muscle made up of two parts: the psoas major and the iliacus. The psoas major begins at the sides of the lumbar spine, then joins with the iliacus when it passes through the back inside surface of the pelvic bowl. Together they pass forward and under the inguinal ligament, at the front of the hip joint, then attaching on the **lesser trochanter** of the femur, a small bump at the top of your inner thigh bone (see Figure 4.3b). In addition to its primary action of hip flexion, the iliopsoas is a slight external rotator of the thigh.

The rectus femoris

The **rectus femoris** is one of the quadriceps group (also see Chapter Five), and the only one of those four muscles that crosses both the knee and the hip joint. It attaches on the upper end to the ilium just below the ASIS, and then below to the patellar tendon, which encircles the patella and attaches to the tibia below the knee. Its action is true hip flexion with no rotation, abduction or adduction added in.

The Assisting Hip Flexors
The sartorius

The **sartorius** (see Figure 4.5) is a long, thin muscle originating on the ASIS and crossing over the thigh to attach to the inner knee. It's a supreme example of the multitasker, moving both the hip and the knee. For the hip, the sartorius is a flexor, an abductor and an external rotator. It moves the bent leg to the side, as in Vrkshasana, *Baddha Konasana* (Bound Angle Pose) and *Sukhasana* (Easy Pose). For the knee, it is a flexor and medial rotator. For safety of the knee, we need to balance that medial rotation with outer rotation of the tibia using the lateral hamstring. In the poses listed above, we would accomplish that by turning the foot and lower leg out. Try one of these poses and feel the muscles mentioned here doing their actions.

The pectineus

The **pectineus** is a very small but strong muscle in the groin. It begins on the upper ramus of the pubic bone, and then attaches on the back of the upper femur. It performs hip flexion along with hip adduction, drawing the leg toward the midline. The arm balance poses require the use of pectineus to hug the legs in onto the arms. (Figure 4.8 shows the pectineus with adductors.)

The tensor fascia lata

The **tensor fascia lata** is a small but very important muscle on the lateral side of the thigh, beginning at the iliac crest and ending in the **iliotibial band**, the strong fascial band that supports the outer thigh and hip. In addition to being a hip flexor, the tensor fascia lata is a hip abductor and medial rotator as well. (Figures 4.5 and 4.10 show the tensor fascia lata.) A special note for yoga alignment: this muscle, despite its small size, is crucial in bringing the top of the thigh back (flexion), turning the thigh inward (internal rotation) and widening it (abduction).

The gluteus medius

The **gluteus medius**, anterior portion, is a broad muscle on the side of the pelvis whose main job is abduction and medial rotation of the hip. It runs from top of the ilium to the greater trochanter of the femur. The anterior portion can assist in flexion. (Figure 4.9b shows the gluteus medius with abductors.) Like the tensor fascia lata, the gluteus medius turns the femur inward, brings it back and widens it. These are important actions for maintaining healthy hip joints.

Poses that strengthen the hip flexors:
Adho Mukha Shvanasana, *Navasana* (Boat Pose), *Padangushthasana* (Toe-Holding Pose) and arm-balance poses.

Poses that stretch the hip flexors:
Virabhadrasana I, Eka Pada Rajakapotasana, *Anjaneyasana* (Deep Lunge Pose) and Urdhva Dhanurasana.

57

The Primary Hip Extensors

The gluteus maximus

The **gluteus maximus**, well-known because it forms the shape of our buttocks, runs from the sacrum diagonally down and across the pelvis to attach into the iliotibial band and the back of the femur. As it extends the hip, it also laterally rotates the thigh. Notice as you take one leg back, either from standing or from Adho Mukha Shvanasana, how easy it is to turn that leg out as it goes back. This is because the fibers of the gluteus maximus run diagonally from the midline out to the side. When we want to keep that back leg parallel, we use the adductor magnus as an antagonist and a stabilizer of the thigh. (See pages 59–60 for the hip adductors.)

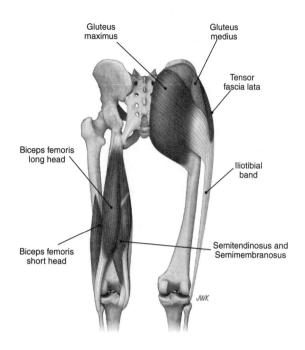

Figure 4.6 *Hip extensors*

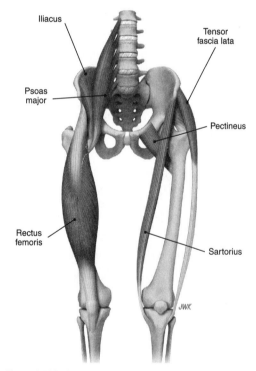

Figure 4.5 *Hip flexors*

The hamstrings

The **hamstrings** are a group of three muscles, all of which originate on the ischial tuberosity, the sitting bone. The lateral hamstring, biceps femoris, attaches on the fibula just below the lateral knee. The **biceps femoris** also has a "short head" (like a sidekick) that originates on the back of the femur bone and then joins the long head to attach below the lateral knee. The two medial hamstrings, **semitendinosus** and **semimembranosus**, are long, thin muscles that attach on the medial tibia, the inner lower edge of the knee. All three hamstrings extend the hip and flex the knee. They can be effectively stretched only when the hip joint is flexed and the knee extended (as in Adho Mukha Shvanasana or all seated forward bends).

If the hamstrings are chronically short and tight, they pull the pelvis into a posterior tilt, which could be detrimental to the hips and the lower back. For more detail, see Chapter Five. The hamstrings are definitely worth getting to know and love!

The Assisting Hip Extensors

The gluteus medius

The **gluteus medius**, posterior portion, can assist in extension, just as the anterior portion of gluteus medius can assist in flexion. In addition to extension, the posterior gluteus medius laterally rotates the femur. (See Figure 4.9a.)

The adductor magnus

The adductor magnus is a large muscle on the inner thigh, attaching at the top to the ischial tuberosity, near the hamstrings' attachment (see Figure 4.7). Its lower attachment is on the center back of the femur bone (on a bony landmark called the **linea aspera**) and on the **medial epicondyle** of the femur, the bony prominence on the inner upper knee. It is a major stabilizer of our gait and posture, and some consider it to be the "fourth hamstring," since its attachments are close to those of the hamstrings. As a member of the hamstring team, the adductor magnus assists in extending the hip joint. We use it in *Setu Bandhasana* (Bridge Pose) to lift the hips (extension) and keep the knees parallel (adduction).

Poses that strengthen the hip extensors: Setu Bandhasana and Urdhva Dhanurasana. Note that the knees are bent, which allows the hamstrings to fully do their work.

Poses that stretch the hip extensors: Supta Padangushtasana and Adho Mukha Shvanasana. Note that the knees have to be straight in order to fully stretch the hamstrings.

In all of the poses named above, we want to do some medial rotation, taking the inner thighs back, and then some lateral rotation, taking the outer thighs back. In both forward bending and backbending, these rotations will recruit the assisting muscles to help guide the femur to be centered in the socket.

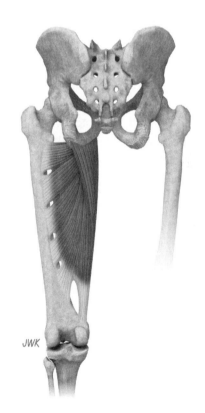

JWK

Figure 4.7 *Adductor magnus*

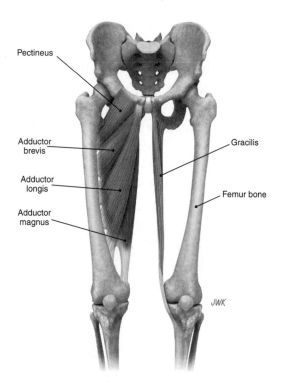

Pectineus

Adductor
brevis

Adductor
longis

Adductor
magnus

Gracilis

Femur bone

JWK

Figure 4.8 *Five adductor muscles*

The Primary Hip Adductors

We have already met a few of these muscles above. The main job of the adductors is to draw the femurs toward the midline, as when you hug your legs onto your arms in *Bakasana* (Crow Pose) or cross your legs in *Gomukhasana* (Cow Face Pose) and Garudasana (see Figure 4.8). Besides that, they are important isometric stabilizers of the thigh, even when the legs do not move toward the midline, as we will see. However, note that they cannot widen the thighs due to their attachment points and angle of pull.

Beginners should note especially the smallest (pectineus) and largest (adductor magnus).

The pectineus

The **pectineus** (which you met before as an assisting flexor) is a very small but strong muscle deep in the groin. It begins on the upper ramus of the pubic bone (the upper wing) and attaches on the back of the upper femur. It performs hip flexion along with hip adduction, drawing the leg toward the midline. The arm balance poses require the use of pectineus to hug the legs onto the arms.

The adductor brevis

The **adductor brevis** runs from the inferior pubic ramus (lower wing of the pubic bone) to the top third of the linea aspera, the bony ridge on the posterior femur.

The adductor longus

The **adductor longus** runs from the inferior pubic ramus to the middle third of the linea aspera. You can easily feel the large tendon of adductor longus in the groin if you adduct your thigh.

The adductor magnus

The **adductor magnus**, mentioned above as an assistor in flexion and extension, begins on the inferior ramus of the pubis and attaches broadly to the linea aspera (back of the femur) and the inner upper knee. You could think of it as the team leader of the adductors.

The gracilis

The **gracilis** is the most superficial and medial of the adductors. It runs from the inferior ramus of the pubis to the inner knee, being the only adductor to cross the knee joint. When you do a pose like Upavishtha Konasana vigorously, you can feel gracilis clearly stretching.

Poses that strengthen the adductors: Any balance pose, any arm-balance pose, Gomukhasana and Garudasana.

Poses that stretch the adductors: Any pose with the legs wide apart, such as Utthita Trikonasana, *Prasarita Padottanasana* (Wide-Leg Forward Bend) and Upavishtha Konasana.

The Primary Hip Abductors

The gluteus medius

The **gluteus medius** (which you have met before, since it is a multitasker) attaches to the top of the ilium, in a broad span from front to back (ASIS to PSIS; see Figure 4.9a). If you put your hands on your hips, you are touching its origin. It then angles down and narrows to attach to the lateral portion of the greater trochanter, the round bony point at the side of your hip.

As mentioned above, this muscle is our main abductor, pulling the femur away from the midline, as in Ardha Chandrasana, but different segments of it can perform other tasks. The anterior portion can flex and medially rotate, and the posterior portion can laterally extend and rotate. It is similar to the deltoid in the shoulder, being large enough to do opposite actions with its outer portions, while

its main action is taking the leg to the side.

When we widen the pelvis and upper thighs, even if the feet do not move apart, we are using this muscle strongly. We do this in Tadasana to provide space for the sacrum. This is the primary muscle that performs "thighs out" in the "shins in, thighs out" action (see page 81 in Chapter Five).

The gluteus minimus

The **gluteus minimus** is a smaller muscle under the gluteus medius (see Figure 4.9b). It has all the same actions but with a smaller range.

The tensor fascia lata

The tensor fascia lata is a small muscle originating on the iliac crest and then attaching into the top of the iliotibial band, which is

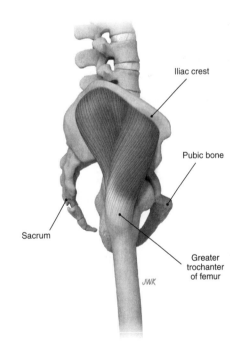

Iliac crest

Pubic bone

Sacrum

Greater trochanter of femur

JWK

Figure 4.9a *Gluteus medius*

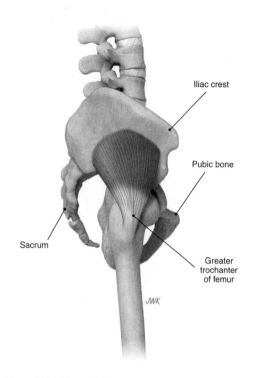

Figure 4.9b *Gluteus minimus*

also called the fascia lata (see Figure 4.10). As you can see from its name, one of its roles is to create tension in the fascial band that supports the outer hip. Its other actions are flexion and medial rotation (since it is located more to the front).

The Assisting Hip Abductors

The sartorius

The **sartorius** is a multitasker that flexes the hip, brings the thigh to the side (abduction) and turns the thigh out (lateral rotation). It runs from the ASIS to the inner lower knee. We use the sartorius to move into Sukhasana and Baddha Konasana (see Figure 4.5).

The piriformis

The piriformis, primarily a lateral rotator (see below), has some capacity to assist in abduction (see Figure 4.11a).

We use the abductors for balance whenever we stand on one foot, even in walking. In yoga methodology, the instruction is often given to bring the tops of the thighs in, back and apart. Note that the little muscle tensor fascia lata performs all of those actions, with help from the other abductors, especially the gluteus medius.

Poses to strengthen the abductors: Ardha Chandrasana and any standing pose in which you isometrically widen your thighs away from the midline such as Uttanasana.

Poses that stretch the abductors: Gomukhasana and the back leg in Utthita Trikonasana.

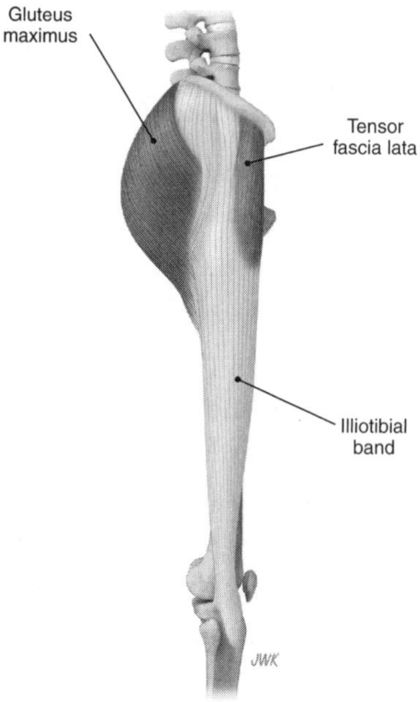

Figure 4.10 *Tensor fascia lata*

The Three Medial Rotators

You're in luck! These three muscles are the same as the three primary hip abductors, so there is no additional list to learn. The attachments of the three abductors on the front (anterior) side of the greater trochanter allow them to turn the femur toward the midline. They are assisted by the anterior portion of the **adductor magnus** (see pages 59–60).

Poses that strengthen the medial rotators: Virasana and any seated pose that has Virasana legs.

Poses that stretch the medial rotators: Baddha Konasana, Utthita Trikonasana, Garudasana and Eka Pada Rajakapotasana.

The Primary Lateral Rotators

These are listed from top to bottom, superior to inferior.

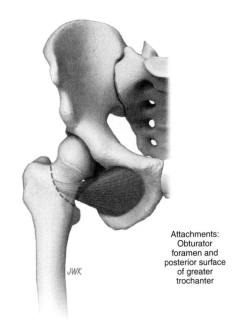

Attachments:
Obturator
foramen and
posterior surface
of greater
trochanter

Figure 4.11b Obturator externus

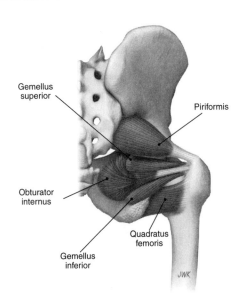

Gemellus
superior

Piriformis

Obturator
internus

Quadratus
femoris

Gemellus
inferior

Figure 4.11a Five lateral rotators

Note that all the lateral rotators attach to the back (posterior) surface of the greater trochanter, in order to pull it back and laterally rotate the thigh. They all stabilize our balance when we stand on one leg. If you want to reduce the list, prioritize piriformis and quadratus femoris.

- The **piriformis** is a small muscle that begins behind the sacrum and travels laterally to reach the top outer portion of the greater trochanter. It is significant for two reasons. First, the sciatic nerve emerges behind it or sometimes through it, which means that tightness in the piriformis can cause sciatic pain. Second, in partnership with the iliopsoas in front, the piriformis stabilizes

63

us in a front-to-back direction (sagittally) when we stand on one foot.

- The **gemellus superior** runs from the ischium to the greater trochanter.

- The **obturator internus** runs from the obturator membrane (fascia inside the obturator foramen) to the greater trochanter.

- The **gemellus inferior** runs from the ischium to the greater trochanter. The two gemellus muscles surround and support the larger obturator internus.

- The **obturator externus** also begins at the obturator membrane and attaches to the greater trochanter (see Figure 4.11b).

- The **quadratus femoris** originates on the lateral side of the ischial tuberosity (sitting bone) and attaches just below the greater trochanter.

The Assisting Lateral Rotators
See above for details on these muscles.

- Gluteus maximus (See Figure 4.6)

- Sartorius (See Figure 4.5)

- Iliopsoas (See Figure 4.5)

Poses that strengthen the lateral rotators: Lateral standing poses like Virabhadrasana II and Parshvakonasana.

Poses that stretch the lateral rotators: Virasana and *Triang Mukhaikapada Paschimottanasana* (Seated Forward Bend with One Leg in Virasana).

The Pelvic Floor
The four bony corners of the pelvic floor are the two sitting bones, the pubic bone and the coccyx. What is often called the pelvic floor or "pelvic diaphragm" is a complex structure of ligaments, fascia and muscles that controls our sphincters and urogenital functions. We will limit our list to three primary muscles (see Figure 4.12). In addition to those listed here, two of the lateral rotators of the hip function as part of this structure (piriformis and obturator internus).

- The **deep transverse perineal** runs from side to side across the pelvic floor, from one inferior ischial ramus to the other. It's not shown here because it's deep to the others listed here. ("Deep

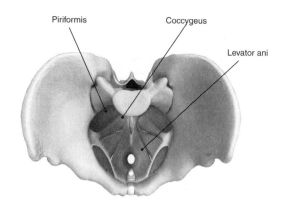

Figure 4.12 *Pelvic floor muscles*

to" is anatomy terminology—"anatomy speak" is what I like to call it—that tells you which muscle is underneath, or deep to, another muscle.)

- The **coccygeus** runs from the coccyx to the ischial tuberosities (diagonally forward).

- The **levator ani** runs between the lower sacrum and the pubic bone (front to back).

These muscles are active when we perform *Mulabandha* (Root Lock), toning and lifting the entire pelvic floor. We need the pelvic floor muscles when we are balancing in any position.

Try this now.
Pick any balancing pose and feel what it's like to do it with and without pelvic floor support.

The Muscles Supporting the Sacroiliac Joint

There are no muscles that directly span across the S-I joint, in contrast with most other moveable joints in the body. When considering muscles to strengthen and stretch for sacroiliac health, include these muscles:

- The quadratus lumborum attaches to the upper rim of the ilium.

- The erector spinae attaches into the lumbar fascia, which is adjacent to the S-I joint.

- The piriformis runs just below the S-I joint, from behind the sacrum over to the greater trochanter of the femur.

- The iliopsoas passes in front of the S-I joint without attaching to the bones. If tight, it could cause compression.

- The gluteus medius and maximus attach to the ilium very close to the S-I joint.

- The transversus abdominus provides indirect support from the sides and front.

- The hamstrings, if tight, will pull the pelvis into posterior tilt, which could strain the S-I joint.

Muscles Used in Basic Yoga Actions

Bringing the femurs and sitting bones back and apart:

- The adductor team stabilizes the femurs.

- The medial rotator team turns the femurs in.

- The flexor team brings the top thighs back.

- The abductor team (gluteus medius, tensor fascia lata) widens the upper thighs.

Note: The adductors are not able to widen the thighs.

Lengthening the sacrum and tailbone:

- The extensor team (gluteus maximus and hamstrings) brings the pelvis into counter-nutation, or posterior tilt.

- The piriformis pulls the sacrum downward and rotates the femurs externally.

- The coccygeus and levator ani draw the coccyx forward toward the pubis.

- The lower rectus abdominus pulls the pubic bone up.

The Big Picture

To feel the deep muscular and fascial line across the front of your hips, try a High Standing Lunge. (The word "high" is used here to distinguish this pose from the low lunge, in which your hands touch the floor.) Proceed with care or skip this pose if you have hyperlordosis or any spinal condition for which backbending is contraindicated. Be sure to connect with your breath as you go.

1. Step your feet apart from front to back, with your left foot forward and your right foot back, the toes of the right foot tucked under. Both legs are parallel and your back heel is off the floor. Your pelvis faces squarely forward. You can put your hands on a chair or wall to help with balance if needed.

2. Lean forward and widen your upper thighs and hips to align the iliopsoas muscle vertically from the lumbar spine down across the front of the hip. Keep that width and lengthen the lower back by drawing downward through the buttocks and up through the abdomen and back ribs. This action will bring length to the middle part of the iliopsoas.

3. Bring your spine upright, and as you do so, feel the fascial connection from your back ankle and deep calf muscles up through your adductors and quadriceps and into your iliopsoas. The top of the iliopsoas overlaps with the diaphragm deep on the front lumbar vertebrae.

4. Take some deep breaths with your chest lifting, and see if you can feel that upper section of the iliopsoas lengthening. As you look up, the fascial line continues up past the iliopsoas through your front throat to your chin.

5. Repeat on the other side.

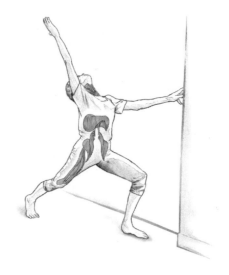

Study Questions

1. Locate the major bones of the pelvis on yourself.

2. What are the six categories of hip-joint movements?

3. What are the two types of pelvic tilt called? What is their significance for spine health?

4. Describe the sacroiliac joint in terms of location, structure and movement.

5. Name at least one muscle from each of the six groups of hip muscles. Why is it useful to know which muscles are multitaskers?

6. Which are your favorite multitasker hip muscles?

7. Which muscle group widens the upper thighs?

8. Name at least one pelvic floor muscle.

9. What muscles overlap in their attachments with the iliopsoas? In other words, which muscles have their attachments near the distal and proximal ends of the iliopsoas?

10. What new things have you learned about the pelvis and hips?

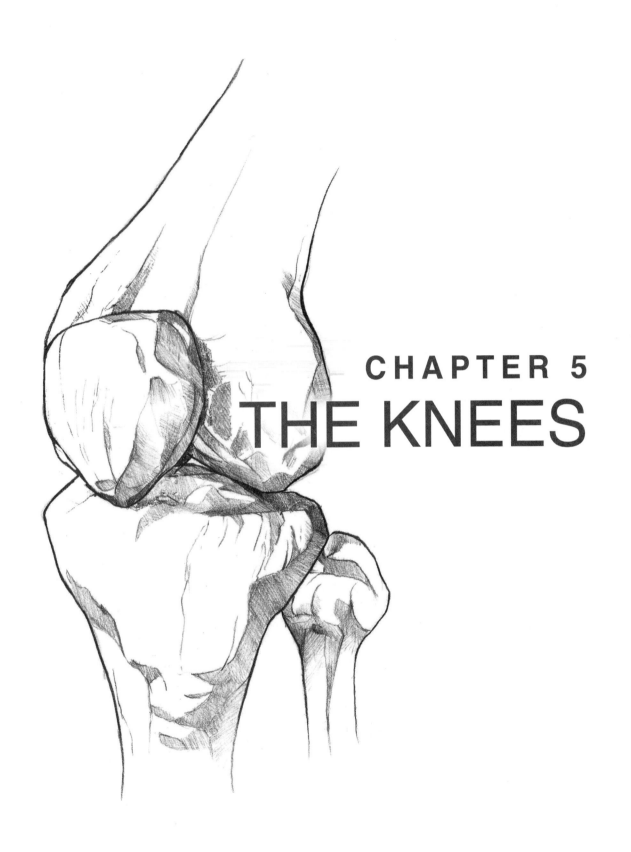

CHAPTER 5
THE KNEES

Take a few steps to really feel the action of your knees. Let them have some spring. Notice the teamwork between the hips, knees and ankles, the fluid coordination that we often take for granted in daily life. With each step, the knees bend and straighten to cushion the impact of our body's weight shifting from one leg to the other. Without them, we'd have no spring in our step, we'd walk like tin soldiers, and we wouldn't be able to jump, or reach to the floor to pick something up, or sit cross-legged on our meditation cushion.

Before we get into the details, here are some basic things to know about the knees.

Because the knees are large weight-bearing joints between very long bones, a great deal of force goes through them when we walk, run, jump or do yoga. Their health depends on the flexibility of the hips and the intelligent alignment of the feet and ankles to help spread and support that load. When the hips or the ankles are very tight, weak or misaligned, the knees will suffer from trying to make up the difference. Given their place between two long bones, the knees are a vulnerable joint.

Knees bend and straighten with very little capacity for rotation. In yoga, we may expect more rotation than they are ready for, as in Virasana or *Padmasana* (Lotus Pose) and all the variations of those poses. In general, to avoid unintended rotations, we point the kneecap in the same direction as the middle toes at all times. Practicing this alignment in standing poses is a crucial part of insuring healthy knees. Also, when doing those poses that could involve rotation in

the knee, be sure to loosen the hips first and approach those poses with care.

Now for the details.

The Bones of the Knee

The femur

The bone at the upper end of the knee is the **femur**, the longest bone in the body (see Figures 4.8 and 5.1). It is shaped somewhat like the number 7, with an angle at the top formed by the **head** (going into the hip joint), the **neck** and the **greater trochanter**, then a long shaft, which is usually not perfectly straight but has a gently bowed shape to give it resilience. The shaft angles inward, allowing for the knee joint to be positioned directly under the hip joint for good weight bearing. At the lower end of the shaft (the distal end, in anatomy speak) are the **femoral condyles** (medial and lateral), which are two large rounded shapes with a hollow gap between them called the **intercondylar notch**. The bottom of the condyles function like the rockers on a rocking chair, allowing the femur to roll over the tibia. In addition to rolling in this hinge-like manner, the femur also glides forward and back across the top of the tibia as we flex and extend the knee. This gliding action increases our range of motion and keeps the femur positioned directly over the tibia during that range.

The tibia

The **tibia**, or shin bone, is the larger of the two bones in the lower leg, continuing the weight-bearing team from the hips to the feet. Its top end, called the **tibial plateau**, is very broad and shaped like a shallow two-part saucer that holds the condyles of the femur. Like the femur, it has **medial** and **lateral condyles** that act as buttresses to hold the weight of the upper body. There is a prominent mound in front called the **tibial tuberosity**, which touches the floor when we kneel or sit in Virasana. You can easily feel it on yourself. The long shaft of the tibia ends with an enlarged prominence on the medial side called the **medial malleolus** (see Figure 6.2a), which is the inner ankle bone. The rest of the distal end forms the top of the ankle joint, joining with the **talus** (see Figure 6.1) a tarsal bone of the foot.

Try this now.

1. Feel the femoral and tibial condyles (the rounded bony prominences above and below the sides of the knees) and the tibial tuberosity just below the knee in front. The long tibia bone is very exposed in the front; you can feel its sharp contour easily on your own leg.
2. Starting at the tibial tuberosity, follow the bone down to the medial malleolus.
3. Go back to the top of the tibia again, and see if you can feel the side edges of the tibial plateau. It will feel like a small groove between the tibia and the femur. This is your actual knee joint.

The patella

The **patella**, or kneecap, is not technically part of the knee joint proper; it is classified as a **sesamoid bone** that floats in connective tissue, which in this case is the tendon of the large quadriceps muscles. Because it can be used as a reference point to work on alignment, we will consider the patella to be part of the knee joint here. Its shape is roughly circular, with a convex outer surface. The undersurface, which fits over the femur and tibia, has ridges, matching the indentations of the other two bones, allowing the patella to glide over the surface of the front of the knee when it bends and straightens. Its function is to protect the front of the knee joint and to provide greater leverage for the four quadriceps muscles whose combined tendon surrounds it (see Figure 5.9). When the four quadriceps muscles develop evenly, the patella "tracks" well in its groove. If one of the quadriceps is weaker or stronger than the others, this tracking becomes imbalanced and causes irritation, known as patello-femoral syndrome.

Try this now.

1. Contract your quadriceps and watch the patella move up and down. Does it travel straight up and down, or at a slight angle?
2. Manually move the patella from side to side with the quadriceps relaxed. This shows you how it is encased in the tendon of the quadriceps.

The fibula

The **fibula** is like an extra buttress under the outer side of the knee, nestled under the lower edge of the lateral tibial condyle and extending down to form the **lateral malleolus** of the ankle (see Figure 6.2a). The fibula is not technically part of the knee joint, but it can rotate slightly, causing changes in the overall alignment of the knee. There is an **interosseous membrane** between the tibia and the fibula, which stabilizes their relationship and provides an attachment site for a few muscles, as well as a division between the compartments of muscles on the back and front of the lower leg.

Try this now.

1. Find the head of the fibula, just below the outer knee.
2. Flex your foot, touching the floor only your heel, and turn your foot in and out. Feel the muscles on the outer calf contracting and the head of the fibula rotating.

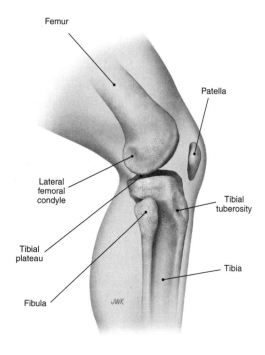

Figure 5.1 *Bones of the knee*

The Support Structures of the Knee and Their Vulnerabilities

The menisci

The **menisci** (singular: **meniscus**, which means "crescent" in Latin) are semicircular cartilage structures that create a cushion, a supportive outer rim on the tibial plateau, and a more secure "seat" for the femoral condyles. They are thicker on the outer edge and thinner at the center, creating a deeper indented shape to stabilize the rounded shape of the distal femur and distribute its weight onto a larger area. The femur sitting on the tibia with the support of the menisci around the edges is like a cup with a rounded bottom sitting in a saucer, rather than on a flat surface (see Figure 5.3). Though the menisci can move slightly in response to knee movements, they can also be torn by forceful twisting. Forcing one's legs into Padmasana without sufficient hip flexibility will cause excessive rotation at the knee, injuring the menisci (see below, Range of Motion).

Common alignment variants: Long-term wear and tear of the menisci can occur with prolonged medial or lateral rotation of the tibia. This rotation may show on the surface as inwardly or outwardly facing patellae. Medial rotation of the tibia is very common in young people, but if it persists through a career in sports, dance, martial arts or yoga, the dangers to the menisci increase.

The collateral ligaments

The collateral ligaments (medial and lateral) run vertically from the femur to the tibia

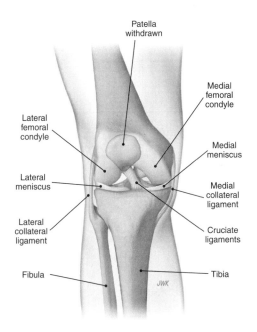

Figure 5.2 *Right knee joint anterior view*

(medially) and the fibula (laterally). Their job is to stabilize the knee in a side-to-side direction. The medial collateral is stronger, and also attached to the medial meniscus, which means that when the medial collateral ligament is injured, the medial meniscus usually is injured as well. These ligaments are taut when the knee is straight and lax when it is bent. For this reason, attempts to improve alignment of the knee are easier when the knee is bent. For the same reason, those recovering from injury will be more stable in straight-legged standing poses than in bent-leg poses, but bent-leg poses will allow for more refined proprioceptive learning.

The cruciate ligaments

The **cruciate ligaments** (anterior and posterior) are inside the joint space, forming a cross from front to back. They prevent

the femur and tibia from shifting forward and back in relation to each other. They are named by their attachment to the tibia; the anterior cruciate runs from the anterior tibia to the posterior femur, and the posterior cruciate runs from the posterior tibia to the anterior femur. They are also positioned obliquely medial to lateral (i.e., not straight anterior to posterior), which allows for flexion of the knee.

Anterior cruciate ligament (ACL) tears are commonly associated with very active sports that involve fast weight shifts, such as soccer and skiing. One assessment of an ACL injury involves what is called a "drawer test," where the assessor attempts to pull the tibia forward in relation to the femur, as in opening a drawer. Laxity in these ligaments could be part of the cause of hyperextension in the knees, in which the top of the tibia moves back beyond the weight-bearing

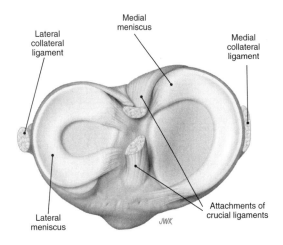

Figure 5.3 *Menisci of the knee (superior view)*

median line of the leg when viewed from the side (See Figure 5.6).

Bursae

There are many bursae around the knee joint, providing spacers between tendons and bone (see Figure 5.4).

Three common anatomical variants

Two common variants of knee alignment are genu valgus ("knock knees") and genu varus ("bow legs"). I like to describe genu valgus as "X legs," meaning that the legs look like the letter X, and genu varus as "O legs" meaning that the legs look like the letter "O" (see Figure 5.5). These conditions are the result of several factors: the anatomical width of the pelvis, the angle of the femur and possibly the uneven length of the collateral ligaments. Depending on the

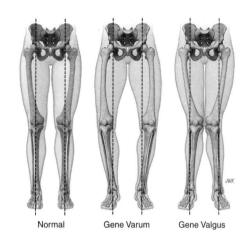

Normal   Gene Varum   Gene Valgus

Figure 5.5 *X legs and O legs*

severity of the deviation, improvements are possible and worthwhile, using the principle of first stabilizing the ankles and shins, then widening the thighs. This muscular action uses a combination of ankle muscles (see eversion in Chapter Six) and hip abduction (see Chapter Four), and yet the benefits go to the knees. We will return to this point (see Yoga Technique Tips later in this chapter).

The third common variant of knee alignment is hyperextension of the knee, when the knee joint (when viewed from the side) is behind the plumb line from the hip to the ankle (see Figure 5.6). This variant can be caused by the structure of the connective tissue (too loose at the back), imbalance of muscles around the knee (weakness of the gastrocnemius muscle) or a genetic formation of the bones of the knee.

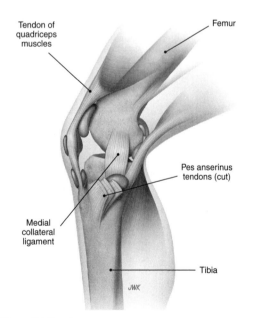

Tendon of
quadriceps
muscles

Femur

Pes anserinus
tendons (cut)

Medial
collateral
ligament

Tibia

JWK

Figure 5.4 *Knee bursae*

Try this now.

1. Experiment with deviations of knee alignment in standing with straight legs, then standing with bent legs.

2. Picturing the placement and function of these support structures, hypothesize and feel the effects of poor alignment: medial rotation of the tibia, hyperextension of the knees, and X legs and O legs.

Range of Motion of the Knee and Yoga Applications

Before we look at the muscles, we will briefly name the ranges of motion of the knee, with associated yoga poses.

If you are just beginning your study of anatomy, you can think of the knee as a hinge, bending (flexion) and straightening (extending, which in this case is returning to neutral from flexion). As much as possible,

align the center of the patella over the center of the toes as you bend your knee. This is called "tracking," and it will train the knees to hinge safely. For beginners, establishing this pattern early in your yoga career is a worthwhile effort.

If you are ready for a more nuanced view of the knees, consider the following smaller ranges of motion.

The glide

As we bend a knee, the distal end of the femur glides forward on the tibial shelf. As we extend the knee, it glides back again. To aid that movement in yoga, we can think of extending forward through the femur bone as we flex, as in poses like Virabhadrasana II and Parshvakonasana. Look at Figure 5.1, and picture the glide of the femur over the tibia.

Rotations

Because the femoral condyles are not equal in size, the femur rotates a small amount as it goes through flexion and extension. Picture a stick with two balls on the end, one ball bigger than the other. If you hold the stick vertically and roll it forward and back on the balls, the stick will turn a bit as it rolls because of the uneven size of the balls. This is the effect when we flex and extend the knee. In flexion the femur rotates laterally and in extension it rotates medially. This is an advantage in poses like Virabharasana II and Parshvakonasana, both of which require lateral rotation and flexion.

Virasana, however, demands medial rotation of the femur with the knee flexed.

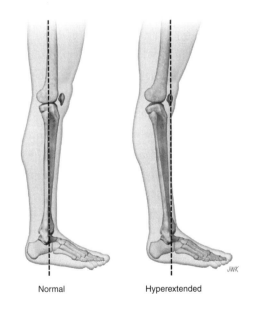

Normal   Hyperextended

Figure 5.6 *Hyperextension of the knee*

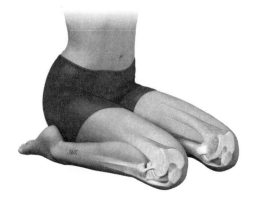

Figure 5.7 *Virasana*

In other words, to bring the foot outside the hip joint in Virasana (see Figure 5.7), we must medially rotate the knee joint a little. If the top of the thigh (at the hip joint) cannot medially rotate enough, the knee will bear the brunt of the demand, and injury to the medial meniscus or medial collateral ligament may result. Manual manipulation of the soft tissue of the thigh can help to ease the strain in this pose. My favorite manual technique is to roll the upper inner thighs back and apart, creating medial rotation in the hip, then roll the lower hamstrings (just above and behind the knee) slightly toward the midline. You can try this and see how it feels in your legs. Each person might need a slightly different manual adjustment according to the bony and soft tissue structure, so I recommend trying different techniques and trusting your evaluation of what works best for you or your student. The goal is to be able to sit in these poses without pain in the knee joint—pain

that feels different from an intense stretch in the muscles.

At the other extreme, Padmasana demands some lateral rotation of the knee in order to bring one foot up onto the opposite thigh (see Figure 5.8). This attempt could strain the lateral collateral ligament if hip range of motion is minimal and the soft tissue in the upper thigh is restrictive. For a student whose knees are higher than the level of the iliac crest when sitting in Sukhasana, Padmasana is a dangerous pose. Eager students may try to pull their foot up onto the thigh without regard to the knee's vulnerability. Those students should not attempt Padmasana, but should work on increasing the needed range of motion in the hip and knee little by little, with poses such as Eka Pada Rajakapotasana with blanket support and the following technique.

Try this now.

1. You can work on gradual external rotation of the knee by sitting high up on a few folded blankets, with one leg in Sukhasana and the other leg out to the side in an easeful position.

2. Place a folded blanket or block under the shin of the bent leg (not the foot) and gradually coax the thigh into more outer rotation.

3. You can supplement the effect of the padding by manually rotating the calf muscle upward and toward you. Also see the section on ankle eversion in Chapter Six for more discussion of this.

The central concept in these examples (one of medial rotation and one of lateral rotation) is to spread the rotation along the whole leg, rather than putting all the demand for rotation only in the knee itself. If you experience pain while attempting these poses, immediately back off and do preparations instead. Forcing the knees will damage them, and they are unforgiving joints.

Having addressed the dangers of these extreme poses, I also must mention the advantage of these poses for joint health: In extreme positions of the knee, the synovial fluid is circulated to the outer corners of the joint space, helping to nourish the cartilage that lines the bones throughout the joint. With regular perfusion of fluids, the cartilage is more likely to remain healthy for a lifetime.

The Muscles of the Knee

For beginners, two large groups of muscles in the thigh (back and front) plus one large muscle of the calf are crucial to know. These are the first three listed below. You can learn the names of muscles within each group, or simply the group's name, location and actions.

The quadriceps

The **quadriceps** are a group of four muscles on the front thigh whose distal (lower) end is a large combined tendon surrounding the patella and attaching to the tibial tuberosity (see Figure 5.9). Their job is knee extension, straightening the knee to return from flexion. Extend your knee right now and watch your muscles contract, the patella move up and the knee become straight. We strengthen

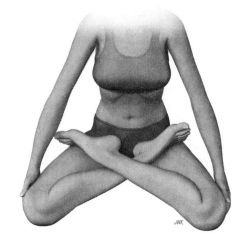

Figure 5.8 *Padmasana*

the quadriceps in all standing poses, and we stretch them in poses like *Supta Virasana* (Reclining Hero Pose).

Here are the names of the four muscles and their upper (proximal) attachments. Only one of them attaches above the hip socket (thereby joining the hip-flexion team), but the others all begin at the upper end of the femur and only cross the knee.

- The rectus femoris is the most superficial muscle, and it does double duty as a knee extensor and hip flexor. Its proximal attachment is the anterior inferior iliac spine, a small bump on the front of the ilium, just above the hip socket. When you begin to lift your thigh, you can feel its tendon pop to the surface. The distal end joins into the patellar tendon.

- The vastus intermedius ("vastus" means "immense" in Latin) begins on the upper front of the femoral shaft and lies underneath the rectus femoris, joining into the patellar tendon.

- The vastus lateralis begins on a prominent ridge at the back of the femur called the linea aspera and wraps around to the front on the outer thigh to join into the patellar tendon.

- The vastus medialis also begins on the linea aspera at the back of the femur and wraps to the front on the inner thigh, also joining into the patellar tendon.

Try this now.

1. Extend your knee strongly and feel the vastus lateralis and vastus medialis. How far around to the sides are they?
2. Watch the large quadriceps tendon (composed of all four muscles together) move the patella up and down.
3. To note the difference between the three quadriceps that cross only the knee and the fourth that also crosses the hip, sit in Virasana. When your spine is upright and your knees are fully flexed, as in Virasana, you are stretching the three vastus muscles that cross only the knee. When you begin to lean back, moving your hips into extension, you also stretch the rectus femoris.

The hamstrings

The **hamstrings** are three muscles at the back of the thigh with a double action: they are hip extensors (bringing the thigh back behind you) and knee flexors (bending the knee). Think of the poses Setu Bandhasana or *Dhanurasana* (Bow Pose) as examples of hamstring strengtheners. We stretch the hamstrings in forward-bending, hip-flexing poses like Adho Mukha Shvanasana and Uttanasana. All three hamstring muscles (minus half of the first one) begin at the sitting bone, the **ischial tuberosity** (see Figure 5.10).

- The biceps femoris has two heads. The longer head begins at the ischial tuberosity, and the shorter head begins on the shaft of the femur. The biceps femoris attaches below the outer knee on the top of the fibula. In addition to its function as a hip extensor and knee flexor, it can rotate the lower leg laterally just a bit, due to its slightly diagonal orientation from top to bottom. This is partly why our knees tend to turn out

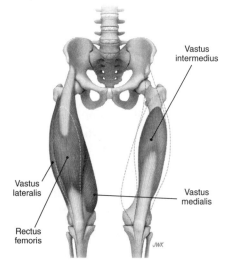

Figure 5.9 *Quadriceps muscles*

when we perform Urdhva Dhanurasana. (The other culprit in that situation is the piriformis muscle; see Chapter Four).

- The semimembranosus runs from the ischial tuberosity down to below the inner edge of the knee, on the upper part of the medial tibia, slightly to the back side.

- The semitendinosus is very close to the semimembranosus, running from the ischial tuberosity down to below the inner knee, slightly toward the front side.

The two inner hamstrings can balance the outer rotation from the biceps femoris by adding a little inner rotation, along with their buddy the adductor magnus (see Chapter Four).

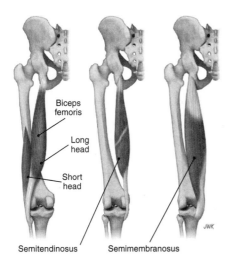

Figure 5.10 *Hamstring muscles*

Try this now.
1. Sit with your knee bent and your foot flexed with only the heel on the floor.
2. Put one hand on each side of the back of your thigh.
3. Pull your heel isometrically back against the floor with your foot turned inward to feel the two "semis" contract, and then with the foot turned out to feel the biceps femoris contract.

The gastrocnemius

The **gastrocnemius** (in Greek, *gastro* means "belly" and *nem* means "leg") is a large muscle in the lower leg that flexes the knee and also plantar flexes the ankle (pointing the foot, see Chapter Six for more about that). Its upper attachment is a two-part tendon attaching above the knee, half going to the medial femoral condyle and the other half to the lateral femoral condyle (see Figure 5.11). Its lower attachment is the Achilles tendon, behind the ankle. We strengthen this muscle in bent-knee poses such as Dhanurasana, and we stretch it in straight-leg poses such as Adho Mukha Shvanasana.

Try this now.
1. To feel the gastrocnemius contract, touch the back of your lower leg.
2. Place your foot on the floor with your knee bent.
3. Slightly lift your heel off the floor, then pull your foot back isometrically toward you. Feel the large "leg belly" do its thing.

That concludes the basic list of the most important knee muscles. For those who want to go further, here are some other interesting elements of the knee joint (two muscles and one common tendon).

- The **popliteus muscle**, the deepest muscle of the knee, runs diagonally across the back of the knee, attaching to the lateral femoral condyle and the upper inner tibia (see Figure 5.12). When it contracts, it medially rotates the tibia in relation to the femur. Its main claim to fame in the muscular teamwork of the knee is that it "unlocks" the knee from extension into flexion.

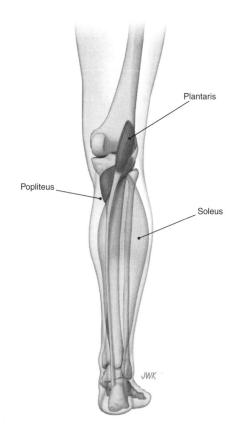

Figure 5.12 *Plantaris and popliteus muscles*

- The **plantaris muscle** has the distinction of having a very small belly but the longest tendon of any muscle in the body (see Figure 5.12). Its belly parallels the larger, deeper popliteus, running diagonally from the outer femoral condyle toward the inner knee, but its tendon extends all the way down to join into the Achilles tendon behind the ankle. You can feel it at the back of the knee, between the two gastrocnemius tendons. It medially rotates the knee and assists in knee flexion.

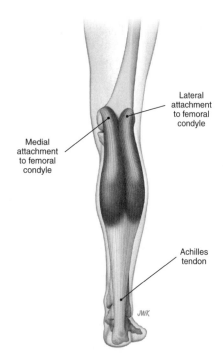

Figure 5.11 *Gastrocnemius muscle*

- The **pes anserinus** is a tendon structure worth knowing, since it is a frequent cause of knee discomfort in yogis. Its name means "goose's foot" in Latin, and it is composed of the combined tendons of the sartorius, gracilis and semitendinosus muscles, attaching to the inner leg just below the knee (see Figure 5.13). It can become irritated when the knee is not aligned properly in any pose.

Yoga Technique Tips

When the hamstrings and the quadriceps are very short and tight, the knee joint will become compressed, which could lead to cartilage or meniscus damage. For students at any level, it is essential to stretch these large muscle groups regularly for the health and safety of the knees. Yoga offers many possible stretches for these muscles, and teachers can creatively and compassionately choose the right stretch for the student's level.

To establish good tracking of the knees, we use a pair of actions called "shins in, thighs out." This double action counteracts the common tendency for the shins to bow out and the thighs to collapse inward toward the midline.

Try this now.

Do the "shins in, thighs out" action and notice the results in your knee alignment.

1. Place a block between your shins and place your feet parallel.

2. Bend your knees, spread your toes and squeeze the block with your lower legs (your inner thighs may contract as well). You are using your peroneal muscles to squeeze the block (see Chapter Six). This is adduction, or movement toward the midline.

3. Keeping that adduction of your lower legs, push your upper legs apart, using the gluteal muscles at the sides of your pelvis to widen the thighs. This is hip abduction. For most people, this will align the knees on the anatomical plumb line, establish good stability in the knees and protect them from injury. It can be used as a therapeutic tool and applied to all poses.

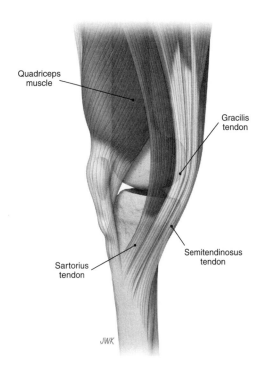

Figure 5.13 Pes anserinus

The Big Picture

To feel the superficial front line of fascia in the lower body, try the pose I call the Wall Quad Stretch. Proceed with care or skip this pose if you have a knee condition or hyperlordosis of the lower spine. Stay in touch with your breath as you explore the pose.

1. Place a blanket on the floor near a wall.

2. Place your right knee on the blanket near the wall and your right foot up the wall in line with the knee. Start with your toes tucked onto the wall (dorsiflexion in the ankle and extension of the toes). Later you can try it with your foot plantar flexed (pointed) on the wall.

3. Step your left foot forward, coming into a lunge facing away from the wall. Lean your upper body forward at first, resting your hands on your left knee to give some slack to the fascial line you are about to stretch.

4. Create tone in the fascial line by pressing your foot into the wall, activating your quadriceps muscle.

5. Keep some of that tone as you begin to bring your torso up to vertical, drawing down through your buttocks and up through your abdomen and your back ribs to keep the lower back spacious. This will bring a strong stretch to your quadriceps muscles of the front thigh.

6. Pull up your lower abdomen, connecting the legs to the torso. Then stretch your front torso up all the way to your collar bones and look up.

7. If you can tolerate more stretch, change the foot that's on the wall to plantar flexion, pointing the toes up the wall.

8. Raise your right arm and look up. You are extending the fascial line of the right side of your front body, including your toe and ankle extensors, quadriceps, rectus abdominis, the fascia of the sternum and the sternocleidomastoids.

9. Repeat on the other side.

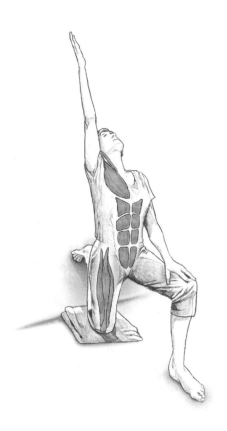

Study Questions

1. Name the bones of the knee, including two that actually form the joint and two that support the joint.

2. Name the three sets of ligaments and cartilage that support the knee, and describe what support they give.

3. Name the front thigh muscle group, with individual muscle names if possible.

4. Name the back thigh muscle group, with individual muscle names if possible.

5. What is the large lower leg muscle that flexes the knee?

6. What is a good basic alignment instruction for the knee in yoga poses?

7. Which types of poses require rotation in the knee, and what are some guidelines for safe practice of these poses?

8. Design a practice for knee health. What poses will you include and why?

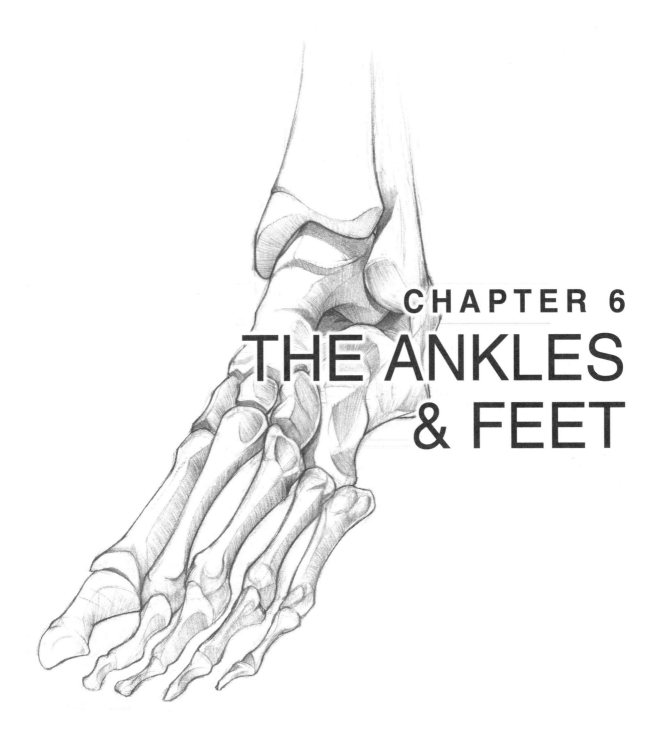

CHAPTER 6
THE ANKLES & FEET

The human foot is a complex structure of 28 bones, over 30 joints and over 20 muscles, all fitting into a relatively small space. As we evolved from four-legged creatures to walking upright, the feet took on more responsibilities. Our feet need to be versatile, providing us with a firm postural foundation and, along with the rest of the legs, the ability to walk, run and dance. The bony structure is strong, yet very mobile, with many small, irregularly shaped bones fitting together like a moveable three-dimensional puzzle. Each foot contains an extensive ligament web that helps us adapt to changing terrain and weight-bearing demands. Like all other parts of the body, the feet will remain healthiest if they are aligned well, and if they move and stretch regularly. Foot and ankle problems develop from leading a sedentary lifestyle, wearing poor shoes, or having poor alignment or movement habits in daily life or exercise. The foot muscles are often weak, even though we usually don't think of them as needing to exercise the way we exercise our backs or our limbs. As we look at the structures of the feet, we will observe what structures give us stability and grounding, and how we can combine that with an energetic lift and resilience. We want to have our feet fully on the ground, yet be free and strong enough to run. The directions of "down" and "up" need to be balanced.

The Bones of the Ankles and Feet

You can feel these bones as we go along.

The Ankle and the Seven Tarsal Bones

The inner ankle bone is the distal end of the tibia, and the outer ankle bone is the distal end of the fibula. These two bones fit like pincers around the sides of one of the tarsal bones called the **talus**, which means "caged bone" (see Figure 6.1). The talus has several curved surfaces where it connects to neighboring bones (tibia, fibula, calcaneus and navicular). It is quite literally a pivotal bone in the foot, serving as a distributor of weight and forces through the foot. Each time we take a step, the talus bone receives the weight of the entire body and passes it forward to the other more distal bones of the foot, toward the toes. Many muscles pass over the talus, yet none attach to it. The top surface is a smooth convex curve called the **trochlea**, allowing the tibia and fibula to roll forward and back over it. (We have a similar trochlear structure in the elbow, another hinge joint.) When the leg bones move forward over the talus, extending the heel as in a pose like Adho Mukha Shvanasana or *Utkatasana* (Chair Pose), we are doing a movement

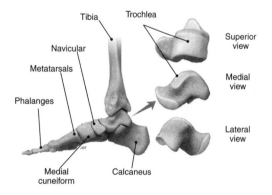

Figure 6.1 Foot bones with three views of the talus bone

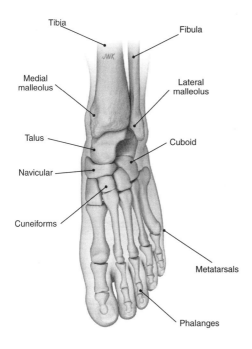

Figure 6.2a Foot bones dorsal view

called **dorsiflexion** in the ankle joint (the **dorsum** is the top surface of the foot; see Figure 6.2a). When the leg bones move backward over the talus, as in pointing the foot in Virasana, we are performing **plantar flexion** in the ankle joint (the **plantar** surface of the foot is the sole; see Figure 6.2b).

Try this now.

1. Sitting with your legs outstretched, move your ankle joints into dorsiflexion and plantar flexion.

2. Picture the rounded top surface of the talus bone providing a curved platform for this movement. Note that this movement is in the sagittal plane, as are all forward- and backward-bending poses in yoga. The only difference is in name: instead of calling it "flexion" and

"extension" as we do in the hip, we call it "dorsiflexion" and "plantar flexion" in the ankle.

Below and behind the talus is the **calcaneus**, or heel bone. Its rounded posterior portion, the tuberosity, is where we first contact the ground when taking a step. Our weight then transfers forward through the rest of the tarsal team: the talus, the large **navicular bone** on the medial side and large **cuboid bone** on the lateral side, and the **three smaller cuneiform bones**, which line up with the first three metatarsals.

The talus has gliding joints (see Figure 1.2) with the calcaneus, the navicular and the cuboid. Multidirectional movements in these joints give us the remarkable ability to

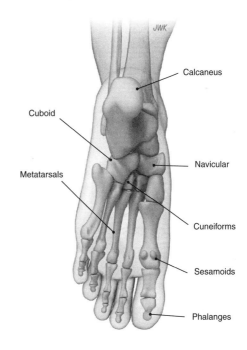

Figure 6.2b Foot bones plantar view

keep our balance while walking on uneven surfaces, and to perform various ankle and foot positions in yoga, such as *Malasana* (Garland Pose) and Prasarita Padottanasana, in which the foot is positioned more medially or laterally in relation to the lower leg. There are four basic types of movements that occur around the talus bone, and you can try them out as you read this next section.

Moving the inner edge of the foot up is called **inversion** (lifting the medial arch), and moving the outer edge of the foot up is called **eversion** (lifting the lateral arch). Perhaps the most common foot misalignment is **pronation**, in which the forefoot (the toe end) abducts (turns out) away from the midline, and the medial arch collapses (extreme eversion). This position puts excessive weight onto the distal end of the first metatarsal, which will gradually enlarge in response, causing a bunion. The contrasting alignment is **supination**, in which the forefoot adducts (turns in) and the medial arch lifts up. Both of these extremes prevent the foot from being an effective foundation for the rest of the body. We can rebalance the foot using the four corners method, described on page 98.

Try this now.
1. Move your foot into inversion, eversion, pronation and supination.
2. Try it without weight, then try it while standing. Send an appreciative thought to your multifaceted talus bone.

The Metatarsals and Phalanges

From the tarsals moving toward the toes, we have five **metatarsal** bones. The metatarsals are long and slender, each with a base that fits into the tarsals, a long shaft, and a head that forms the base of each toe. The first metatarsal (on the big-toe side, since the big toe is also called the first toe) is thicker and stronger, which we need in order to push off with the foot when walking and running. The base of the fifth metatarsal is also larger than the others, providing stability on the outer edge of the feet. You can feel the tuberosity of that bone on the outer side of your foot.

There are two **sesamoid bones** (small, round and "sesame-like") under the head of the first metatarsal that surround and protect the tendon of the flexor hallucis longus (see Figures 6.2b and 6.12). Without these two bones as spacers, that flexor tendon would get excessive wear and tear with each step.

The **phalanges** are the bones of the toes. The same word is used for the bones of the fingers, and the singular form of this word is **phalanx**. The big toe has two phalanges, and the other toes each have three phalanges. They are named by their location: proximal, medial and distal. The joints between each phalanx are hinge joints whose main movements are flexion and extension.

Try this now.
1. Hold a toe and experiment with how much you can move it passively (i.e., moving it with your hand rather than with your toe muscles).

2. Try active movements with each toe separately.

3. Hold the foot with both hands and see how much passive movement you can get between the metatarsals by twisting your foot in your hands. This kind of passive stimulus is good for developing awareness and increasing circulation in the feet.

Before we move on to other topics, take note that the number of bones in the legs progresses from one bone in the femur, then two in the lower leg (tibia and fibula), then three at the ankle (talus, calcaneus and navicular), then four across the mid-foot (cuboid and three cuneiforms), then five metatarsals, then…not six toes, but five toes each made up of a few bones. It's an organized and elegant progression from unity to diversity that is repeated in the arms and hands as well.

The Arches

We have three structural arches in the foot: the longer medial one on the big-toe side, the smaller lateral one just below the outer ankle bone, and a transverse arch across the heads of the metatarsals (see Figure 6.3). These arches are formed and supported by the shapes of the bones and by a web of ligaments and muscles, which are outlined in this chapter. Healthy arches help to absorb the weight of the body and distribute it over the whole foot evenly, and to give us resilience in walking and running. They need to release a bit to receive and respond to our weight, but stabilize to transmit it.

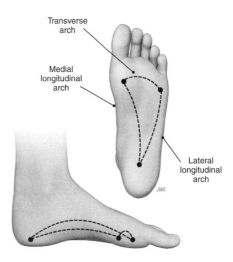

Figure 6.3 *Arches of the foot, plantar and medial views*

If someone has "fallen arches" or "flat feet," they may have very weak foot muscles. Later in this chapter we'll look at some strengthening exercises to help maintain healthy arches.

From a functional viewpoint, we can divide the foot into two parts: medial and lateral (see Figure 6.4). As we step, our weight goes onto the heel. (It's interesting to observe which part of the heel strikes first. For many people, the outer heel strikes first because the leg is naturally turned out. This causes the heels of our shoes to wear out first on the outer edge. We can train ourselves to place the center of the heel down, a better option because it recruits support equally on both sides of the foot, knee and hip.) After the heel, the weight transfers through the talus to the navicular, three cuneiforms, three metatarsals and toes. We push off to propel ourselves forward with the first toe joint, lifting the heel with the triceps surae group of muscles (gastrocnemius and soleus, two muscles you

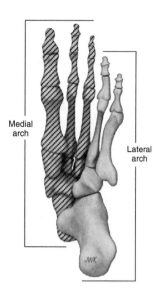

Figure 6.4 Medial and lateral foot

will meet shortly). We use our lateral foot (the cuboid, two metatarsals and toes) less for propulsion and more for balance.

Try this now.
Take a few steps to observe how you transfer weight from your heel to your toes with each step. Note how much movement occurs. Does it go straight along the center line of your foot, or does it curve to one side or the other?

The Connective Tissue of the Feet

Given the relative mobility of the foot, with 28 bones and over 30 joints, the support from ligaments and fascia is particularly important in the feet. There are over 100 ligaments in each foot, some of them very small, of course. We'll focus on a few support structures in particular.

Plantar fascia

The **plantar fascia** spans the whole inferior surface of the foot (see Figure 6.5). Its attachments are the front of the heel (calcaneus) and the base of all five toes (phalanges). This fascia supports the longitudinal arches. When we lift our toes, the fascia is pulled tightly like a bowstring, causing the inner arch to lift up. The plantar fascia depends on the support of plantar ligaments and muscles under the sole of the foot; without that support, the fascia becomes strained and develops tears, resulting in plantar fasciitis. See the end of this chapter for some exercises that help with plantar fasciitis.

Try this now.
1. With some weight on one foot, observe the height of your arch.
2. Lift all five toes, and see how much more the arch lifts. Picture the fascia spanning that entire distance.

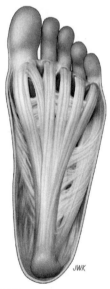

Figure 6.5 Plantar fascia

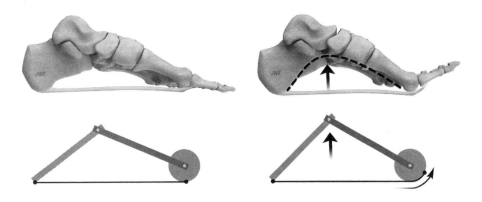

Figure 6.6 *Arch lifting when toes lift*

Ligaments

If you sprain your ankle, it is very likely that what gets injured are the **lateral ligaments**, attaching the lateral malleolus to the talus and calcaneus (see Figure 6.7). On the medial side, a stronger, larger ligament called the **deltoid ligament** and a smaller one called the **spring ligament** protect the inner ankle. There are also two plantar ligaments stabilizing the tarsal and metatarsal bones from below (see Figure 6.8). These structures help to allow for quite a bit of forward-backward movement but also stabilize your ankle from excessive side-to-side movement.

The **retinacula** (singular: **retinaculum**) of the ankle are ribbon-like bands of fascia that wrap around the ankle in order to organize and protect the various tendons, nerves and blood vessels passing over the ankle (see Figure 6.13). We have similar retinacula in the wrist (see Figures 8.5a and 8.12).

The Muscles of the Ankles and Feet

Foot muscles can be divided into two groups: those whose belly is in the lower leg, with long tendons extending into the feet, called the extrinsic muscles, and those that are entirely within the foot, called the intrinsic muscles. Beginning students can focus on group one, then continue on with the other groups when you're ready for more.

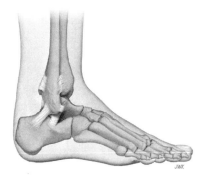

Figure 6.7 *Lateral ankle ligaments*

Group One: The Primary Ankle and Foot Muscles

The gastrocnemius

The **gastrocnemius** is the most superficial muscle on the back of your lower leg (see Figure 6.9). Its two proximal (upper) attachments reach across the back of the knee to connect to the condyles of the femur, fitting between the tendons of the hamstrings. Its distal attachment is the Achilles tendon, inserting onto the calcaneus, or heel bone. It performs flexion of the knee and plantar flexion of the ankle.

The soleus

The **soleus** is deeper and thicker than the gastrocnemius, and it crosses the ankle joint but not the knee (see Figure 6.9). Its proximal attachment is on the upper posterior tibia and fibula, and its distal attachment is also the Achilles tendon. It is considered to be important in pumping blood back to the heart with each step we take. The term **triceps surae** denotes the gastrocnemius and the soleus together. These two muscles do the work of bringing you up onto tiptoe. We use them to stabilize the ankles and feet in yoga. We often need to "iron" them out in order to do a pose with extreme knee flexion like Virasana.

The tibialis anterior

The **tibialis anterior** is at the front of the shin, just lateral to the tibia bone (see Figure 6.10). It runs from the lateral upper tibia, just under the knee, down across the ankle and under the sole of the foot on the inner edge. You can feel its tendon easily, as described below. Its main action is dorsiflexion, with some inversion (inner-arch lifting) added in.

Try this now.

1. Sitting with one foot flat on the floor, lift up your heel. Feel the contraction of the triceps surae muscles at the back of your calf.
2. Place your heel on the floor as you lift the forefoot up, especially the inner arch. You can clearly see and feel the tendon of tibialis anterior as it crosses the ankle joint and the firmness of the muscle along the outer edge of the tibia bone.

The peroneals

The **peroneals** (also called fibularis) are two muscles on the outer edge of the calf that support the outer ankle (see Figure 6.11a and 6.11b). The two muscles are called **peroneus longus** and **peroneus brevis**. They run from the top of the fibula, down across the outer ankle, wrapping under the outer ankle bone and under the sole of the foot.

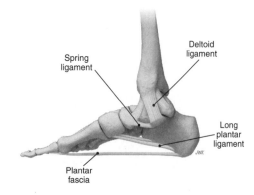

Figure 6.8 *Medial and plantar ligaments*

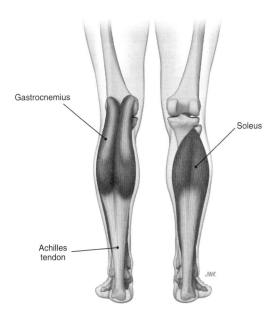

Figure 6.9 *Gastrocnemius and Soleus*

They strengthen the outer edge of the foot, as in Vasishthasana, where we need that outer edge to be a stable foundation, and in the lift of the upper foot in Ardha Chandrasana. We use them to activate the outer edges of the feet in poses such as Eka Pada Rajakapotasana and *Adho Mukha Vrksasana* (Handstand). They are also involved when we push down through the inner heel in any standing pose and when we move the shins toward the midline in the action called "shins in, thighs out" (see Chapter Five).

Try this now.

1. In Adho Mukha Shvanasana, lift your heels high and feel the gastrocnemius and soleus contract to plantar flex your ankle. Notice the difference in muscular use between pressing down more on the little-toe side of your foot as compared to the big-toe side. We'll come back to that later when we analyze the four corners technique.

2. Press the inner heel down toward the floor. Notice the peroneals contracting at the lateral side of your calf, performing eversion.

3. Reach your outer heel down toward the floor. Here it's your tibialis anterior working to perform inversion and dorsiflexion, and you can see and feel its tendon pop up at the front of your ankle. Note how this action lifts your inner arch.

4. Find the place in the middle where both sides of the heel reach down.

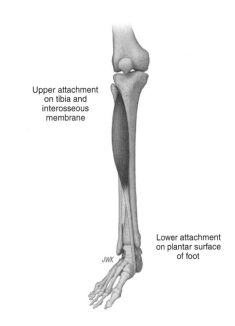

Figure 6.10 *Tibialis anterior*

Group Two: The Deeper Extrinsic Muscles

The tibialis posterior

The **tibialis posterior** is underneath the gastrocnemius at the back of the calf. It begins at the top back portion of the tibia and fibula, and the interosseous membrane between those two bones. Its tendon passes under the medial malleolus (the inner ankle bone) to attach to several tarsal and metatarsal bones under the sole of the foot. It is an important support for the inner arch, especially when the heel is raised in plantar flexion. It activates when we press the mound of the little toe down in any standing pose or in Adho Mukha Shvanasana (see Figure 6.12).

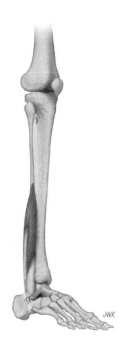

Figure 6.11b *Peroneus brevis*

The toe flexors

The **toe flexors** (one for the big toe, **flexor hallucis longus**, another for the other four toes, **flexor digitorum longus**) press the tips of the toes down, and in the process they also help to support the inner arch, the action of inversion (see Figure 6.12). They have leverage to do that because their tendons curl around the medial malleolus (along with tibialis posterior). These long tendons start at the toes, continue under the sole of the foot and wrap under the medial malleolus. The muscle bellies begin above the ankle, and they insert onto the back of the tibia and fibula.

Note: The flexor hallucis longus is an important part of pushing off from one foot

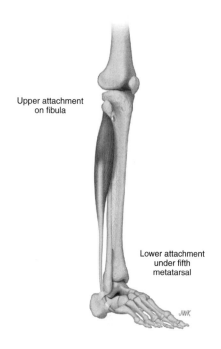

Upper attachment on fibula

Lower attachment under fifth metatarsal

Figure 6.11a *Peroneus longus*

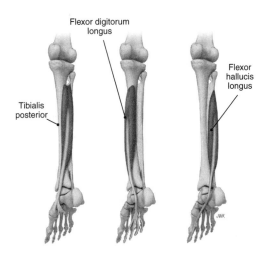

Figure 6.12 *Extrinsic toe flexors and tibialis posterior*

3. Lift your heel and put more weight onto the outer foot, and you'll feel the tibialis posterior contract.
4. Lift all your toes (but not the ball of your foot) and touch the lower front shin, feeling the toe extensors underneath tibialis anterior.

We use these muscles for balance; even a small contraction from one or more of these important stabilizers will shift our balance.

to the other as we step or run. Its tendon is vulnerable to compression between our body's weight and the floor, so we have two small sesamoid bones that surround it and take some of that weight.

The toe extensors

The **toe extensors** (one for the big toe, **extensor hallucis longus**, another for the other four toes, **extensor digitorum longus**) lift the toes up (see Figure 6.13). They begin at the lateral side of the front shin and extend down across the ankle all the way to the toes.

Try this now.
1. Touch the back of your Achilles tendon to feel the tendons on either side of it.
2. Press all five toes down; you'll feel the flexor digitorum longus and flexor hallucis longus contract.

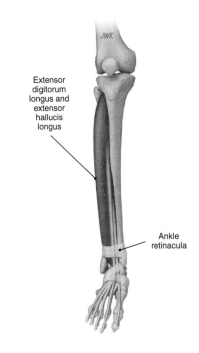

Figure 6.13 *Extrinsic toe extensors*

Group Three: The Intrinsics

There are four layers of intrinsic muscles of the feet, and we will include some of them here. The muscles described below are crucial in supporting the arches, using the toes for balance and aligning the foot. You

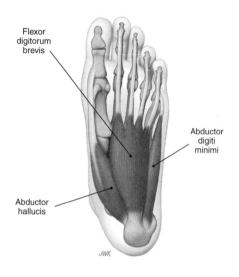

Figure 6.14a *Intrinsic toe abductors and flexors*

will see additional muscles depicted in the illustrations. Hopefully, being aware of these versatile foot muscles might help us to use them wisely!

The abductor hallucis

The **abductor hallucis** brings the big toe away from the other toes. Its belly is at the back end of the medial longitudinal arch, a good position to help lift the arch when we "widen" the big toe (see Figure 6.14a). Its attachments are at the proximal joint of the big toe and the front inner border of the heel. When the big toe deviates inward, as in a bunion, this muscle will weaken. Strengthening it can retard the development of bunions. See suggestions below in the foot exercise section for how to do this.

The abductor digiti minimi

The **abductor digiti minimi** widens the little toe away from the other toes. Its belly extends from the proximal end of the little toe back to the heel. It is a strong supporter of the peroneals in a pose like Vasishthasana, in which we bear weight on the outer edge of the bottom foot.

The flexor digitorum brevis

The **flexor digitorum brevis** extends from the middle phalanx of toes 2–5 back to the front of the calcaneus. As it flexes the toes, it provides a strong support for the plantar fascia and the arches.

The quadratus plantae

The **quadratus plantae** is an important support to the plantar fascia (see Figure 6.14b). It attaches to the front of the heel, then to

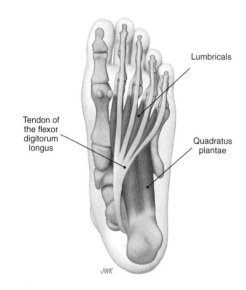

Figure 6.14b *Lumbricals and quadratus plantae*

the tendon of the flexor digitorum longus muscle (note that muscles do not always attach bone to bone!). It assists in flexion of the toes and participates in the "foot shrinking" exercise below.

The lumbricals

The **lumbricals** attach to the divided tendons of the flexor digitorum longus, and then to the proximal phalanx (bone) of toes 2–5. When we contract the lumbricals, it supports the transverse arch in an action that is often called "doming the foot." The toes stay extended, but the base of the toes lifts up.

The dorsal interossei

The **dorsal interossei** are a team of small muscles on the dorsal (top) side of the feet between the metatarsals, with their tendons extending onto the toes (see Figure 6.14d). They spread the toes apart.

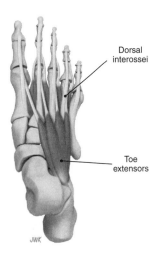

Figure 6.14d *Dorsal interossei and toe extensors*

The plantar interossei

The **plantar interossei** are a similar team of small muscles on the plantar (bottom) side of the feet between the metatarsals, with tendons extending onto toes 3–5 (see Figure 6.14e). They adduct the toes toward each other.

Try this now.

1. Sitting in a chair or standing, place your feet parallel and flat on the floor.
2. Reach down and spread your hands over the tops of your feet, wrapping around to the sides.
3. Looking at our list of intrinsics, use each muscle and feel the movements under your hands. Consider how these muscles contribute to stability and alignment of the feet and of the entire body.

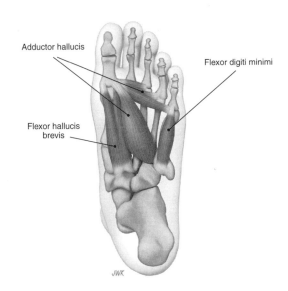

Figure 6.14c *Intrinsic toe adductors and flexors*

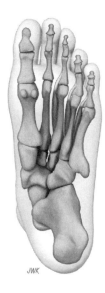

Figure 6.14e *Plantar interossei*

Exercises

The Four Corners Exercise

This exercise is a good way to balance the weight on your feet, and to awaken and strengthen muscles that support the three arches. Good foot alignment makes it possible to support the legs and spine in the best possible way. With weak feet, the chain of collapse continues up the body and can cause many other problems in the knees, hips and spine. It's really worth the effort to establish a good foundation in the feet. I developed this sequence after observing many feet and finding that this sequence helps people to maintain a good foundation in yoga and in daily life. Follow the sequence with one foot and review the muscles

mentioned as you go along (see Figure 6.15). The steps accumulate: you maintain step 1 as you do step 2, on so on. Then of course, repeat on the other foot.

1. Press only the inner heel into the floor, lifting the rest of the foot off the floor. (Muscles used: tibialis anterior and peroneals.)

2. Keeping the inner heel down, press the base of the little toe down. This pathway crosses diagonally over the foot, activating strong extrinsics and intrinsics. (Muscles used: tibialis posterior, gastrocnemius, abductor hallucis, abductor digiti minimi and lumbricals.)

3. Widen across the foot to press the big-toe mound down. (Muscles used: abductor hallucis, abductor digiti minimi, soleus and gastrocnemius.)

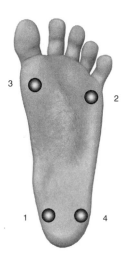

Figure 6.15 *Four corners of the foot*

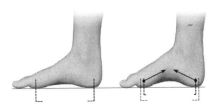

Figure 6.16 Foot shrinking

4. Cross diagonally back to the outer heel. (Muscles used: tibialis anterior, abductor hallucis and quadratus plantae.) This last step gives an extra lift to the inner arch.

When you have done all four corners, notice that you have a strong foundation into the ground, and also a good muscular lift up through your feet and lower legs.

Other Foot Exercises

Foot shrinking

With some weight on one foot, shrink the metatarsals and toes back toward the heel. Do this several times, and notice that you are using both intrinsic and extrinsic muscles. The arch will lift and your toes may also curl a bit (see Figure 6.16). This exercise is beneficial for plantar fasciitis. (Muscles used: quadratus plantae, flexor digitorum brevis and lumbricals.)

Toe curling

Sit in a chair and work one foot at a time. Curl your toes under and sweep them in toward the midline, in a gesture similar to gathering crumbs off the dinner table with your hand. This movement activates the muscles of your arch, particularly the toe flexors and the abductor of your big toe. (Muscles used: flexor digitorum brevis and longus, flexor hallucis longus, tibialis posterior, abductor hallucis, plantar interossei and tibialis anterior.)

The alphabet

Stretch your leg out in front of you while sitting. With your heel staying on the floor, write the alphabet with your foot, picturing the toes as scribes. Feel the multidirectional movements required. This is a standard physical therapy exercise for healing a sprained ankle, and it works all your foot and ankle muscles. For variety, write a message to yourself or someone else, spelling each word carefully with your foot movements.

Everyday habits

Our feet need good shoes for support and protection, but they also need to move. Consider whether the shoes you wear on a daily basis provide enough room in the toe box for your toes to spread, enough support through the arch, and enough movement throughout the shoe for your foot to stretch with each step. If you plunk your whole foot down with each step, falling from foot to foot instead of using the spring of the foot's natural movement, the soft tissue of your feet will gradually weaken and you will lack the support for the rest of your body. Going barefoot whenever you can will help to develop strength and versatility in the muscles of your feet.

Gravity pulls on us 24–7, and when we are standing, our feet have to orchestrate our body's weight and our movements on a comparatively small structure. With knowledge and practice we can refine how we position our bones (the downward component) and also how we engage our muscles (the upward component) in order to achieve strength, stability and mobility for whatever we want to do. The feet provide the foundation for good alignment in the entire body, making them supremely worthy of our attention.

The Big Picture

To feel fascial connections that connect your ankles with the rest of your body, stand on a rolled mat or blanket. The pose described here is Uttanasana, but if you have any contraindication for forward bending, you can remain standing in Tadasana near a wall and still feel a very good stretch of the lower part of the fascial line through your ankles. If you have an ankle injury or plantar fasciitis, use a very small roll. Remember to breathe easefully as you go.

1. Place your metatarsals up on a rolled blanket with your heels on the floor behind the roll. If you are doing Tadasana, touch the wall for support and feel your ankles and calves stretching. If you are doing Uttanasana, fold forward and bring your hands to blocks, a chair or the floor. This exercise involves balance, so I recommend using a chair to support your hands at first.

2. Lift one heel at a time to engage the gastrocnemius and soleus muscles. Then return to touching the floor with both heels.

3. If you are doing Uttanasana, extend your spine forward a bit, toning your hamstrings and spinal extensors.

4. Gradually straighten your knees, bringing your weight forward while still keeping the heels down. Support yourself with your hands, since this variation brings the weight forward more than usual in the pose.

5. After a minute or so, step off the roll and onto the floor, performing Uttanasana the usual way. See if your head lowers further, and if you feel more space in your legs and spine from accentuating the stretch over the back of the ankle.

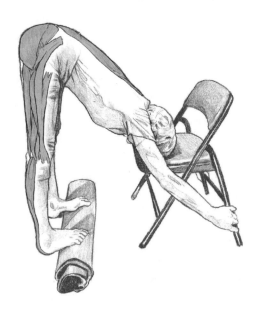

Study Questions

1. Show dorsiflexion, plantar flexion, eversion, inversion, pronation and supination.

2. What bones form the ankle joint? What movements occur here?

3. The seven bones at the hind foot are called the _____.

4. The five long bones distal to those are the _____.

5. The toe bones are called _____.

6. Describe the location and function of the plantar fascia.

7. Describe the location and action of these muscles: tibialis anterior, gastrocnemius, soleus and peroneal group.

8. How is the medial longitudinal arch supported?

9. Examine the many positions of the feet in yoga poses and review what joint actions and muscular support are required for each. Examples: Adho Mukha Shvanasana, Virasana, Malasana, Prasarita Padottanasana, the back foot in Parshvakonasana, the back foot in Virabhadrasana I and the back foot in High Lunge.

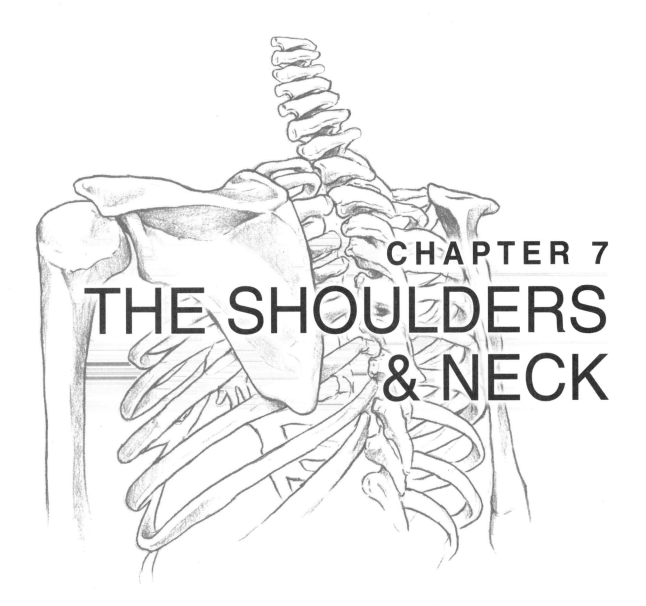

CHAPTER 7
THE SHOULDERS & NECK

It is through our head, neck and shoulders that we interact with the world around us. We perceive our surroundings through four of our five senses centered there (taste, smell, sight and hearing), and the carriage of this part of the body expresses a lot about who we are on the inside. You can probably think of times when you have felt tired, sad, wounded or scared, and your shoulders round forward and your neck shortens. We may comfort ourselves by covering the front of the chest to protect the heart. When we feel happy and expansive, we might hold our head high and our shoulders broad. There are common sayings that involve this part of the body as expressions of inner states, such as "don't carry the weight of the world on your shoulders" and "keep your chin up."

When we consider the Tantric view and see the body as a temple with the heart as its center, the shoulders, neck and head are the pinnacle of the temple, with the potential of expressing tremendous strength and dignity. In asana and pranayama, shoulder alignment is paramount. Collapse in this part of the body restricts our breathing and therefore our vitality. Poor alignment and weakness in the shoulders are the most common causes of many of the pains and strains that afflict yoga practitioners and non-yogis alike. When we understand the structures involved in the shoulders, both strengths and vulnerabilities, we can choose to practice in a way that maintains good alignment and a good balance of stability and freedom. This chapter will outline the shoulder and neck bones, joints and

muscles, and will explore healthy alignment to keep the shoulders and neck fully functional and freely expressive. And yes, we will consider the challenges of Chaturanga Dandasana.

The Shoulder Girdle

The shoulder girdle consists of the **scapula** (shoulder blade), the **clavicle** (collarbone) and the **humerus** (upper arm bone) (see Figure 7.1). The only connection of the shoulder girdle to the trunk of the body (the axial skeleton) is through the **sternum**, or **breastbone**, located in the center front chest. The shoulder girdle floats on the ribs like a cape, embedded in fascia and muscles, with no joint connection to the core of the body other than the **sternoclavicular joint** in the front. Because of this, as we will see, we have a big range of motion with our arms but also some danger of joints and muscles being strained by extreme movements.

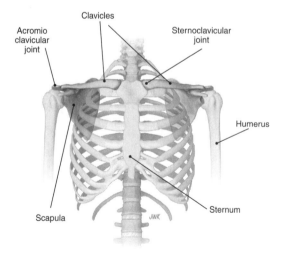

Figure 7.1 Shoulder girdle bones

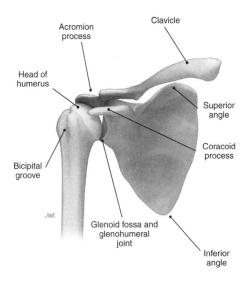

Figure 7.2a Scapula anterior view

The Scapula

The scapula is a roughly triangular bone with uniquely shaped features at the top and the front (see Figures 7.2a and 7.2b). It glides over the upper back ribs, tethered only by its attachment at the front to the sternum (breastbone) via the clavicles (collarbones) and by the many muscles that stabilize and move it from all sides. The landmarks on the scapula are worth knowing as reference points. There is a bony ridge called the **scapular spine** near the top of the scapula, ending in the cap at the top of your shoulder, called the **acromion process**. Just below the acromion process and facing laterally is the **glenoid fossa**, a saucer-shaped surface into which the arm bone fits. This is what's generally known as the "shoulder joint," and its technical name is the **glenohumeral joint**. From its wide top, the scapula narrows down to a point called the **inferior angle**.

At the top end, the **superior angle** (located on the top medial part of the scapula) is hard to feel because there are many muscles over it, but it is worth knowing because of a muscle that attaches to it, the **levator scapulae**. On the front, there is a finger-shaped protrusion called the **coracoid process**, which angles laterally and provides attachment for several muscles we will meet later. You can feel the end of the coracoid process as a small bump just anterior to the humeral head and the shoulder joint.

Note that while the shoulder is considered to be a ball-and-socket joint, the socket is very shallow compared to the hip joint. It's like comparing a bowl with an orange in it (the hip joint) and a spoon with a lime in it (the shoulder joint). This shallow spoon shape makes more movement possible, but the trade-off is that the shoulder has less structural stability and is very dependent on the muscles to stay properly aligned and protected.

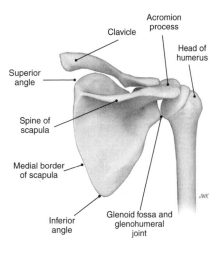

Figure 7.2b Scapula posterior view

The Clavicle

The clavicle is a shallowly S-shaped bone that articulates with the acromion of the scapula laterally (at the **acromioclavicular joint**) and with the sternum medially (at the **sternoclavicular joint**). It is clearly visible on the top front chest. The clavicle provides a horizontal strut that maintains the width of the shoulder girdle and connects the arm and scapula to the core of the body via the sternum. It is the most frequently broken bone in both children and adults.

The Humerus

The **humerus** is the upper arm bone, consisting of a head, a shaft and epicondyles at the lower end, which form part of the elbow joint. Other landmarks include the greater tuberosity and the lesser tuberosity (two protrusions on the sides of the humeral head, which are similar to the trochanters of the femur and are significant in shoulder alignment). Between those tuberosities toward the front is the **intertubercular groove**, also known as the **bicipital groove**, through which the tendon of the biceps muscle passes. Another landmark is the trochlea at the lower end of the humerus, a structure like a rolling pin, which allows the elbow to function as a hinge.

Movements of the Shoulder Girdle

The scapula does the following movements, carrying the humerus along with it:

- Elevation: moving straight up (shrug)

- Depression: moving straight down (pull 'em down!)

- Retraction: moving toward the spine (squeeze them together behind your back)

- Protraction: moving away from the spine, around the sides of the ribs (give a hug)

- Upward rotation: tilting the glenoid fossa upward (reach an arm overhead)

- Downward rotation: tilting the glenoid fossa downward (fold an arm behind your back)

- Posterior tilt: the top of the scapula moves back (stand tall, shoulders back)

- Anterior tilt: the top of the scapula moves forward (hunch forward)

The humerus does the following movements, which may move the scapula as well:

- Flexion: bringing the arm forward

- Extension: bringing the arm back

- Medial rotation: rotating in toward the front midline

- Lateral rotation: rotating away from the front midline

- Abduction (also called horizontal flexion): moving the arm to the side

- Adduction: moving the arm across the front body

Note: To understand the movements of the scapula and humerus, we have isolated each from the other, but this doesn't happen in normal movement. As you do the movements listed below, notice how much more range of motion you have when combining scapular and humeral movement together.

Try this now.
1. Find these bones and landmarks on someone else:

- The clavicles

- Landmarks on the scapula: the acromion, the coracoid process, the spine, the medial border and the inferior angle Note that you can't feel the glenoid fossa or the superior angle, but you can indicate where they are.

- The humeral head and the epicondyles of the humerus

2. Place your hand over a friend's scapula to feel it moving in each direction. When they do a complete circle with their arm, can you feel how much the scapula moves? Note the differences in range of motion between the hip and the shoulder, even though both are ball-and-socket joints.
3. Move your own humerus in each direction listed above, and think of a yoga pose that requires that each movement.

Notice at which point the scapula has to be involved in the movement, especially when the arm goes overhead.

The Connective Tissue of the Shoulder

There are several ligaments at the front of the shoulder girdle connecting the clavicle, coracoid process and acromion. The back of the scapula is secured only by muscles.

Because the shoulder joint has such a large range of motion, it needs a very loose capsule around the joint, and this capsule functions like a kind of ligament. When your arm is hanging down, the top of the capsule is taut and the bottom of the capsule is loose and has numerous folds. Similarly, when you raise your arm overhead, the bottom of the capsule becomes taut and the top of the capsule has extra "fabric" and becomes bunched up. This is an important thing to remember for later when we consider injuries of the shoulder. One common injury, **frozen shoulder** or **adhesive capsulitis**, occurs when the folds at one side of the capsule become "glued" together, making most movements difficult and painful.

To provide a closer fit of the humeral head into the glenoid fossa, there is a ring of cartilage around the circumference of the fossa called the **glenoid labrum**, or lip.

There are bursae in several locations around the shoulder joint, helping to cushion the edges of the bones and allowing for smooth movement of the tendons over each other and over the bones. When the muscles are contracted for long periods of time, these bursae can become inflamed, causing pain.

The Brachial Plexus

Peripheral nerves emerge from the spinal cord at all levels of the spine. The nerves that arise from C1-4 serve the head and neck. The nerves that arise from C5-T1 are collectively called the **brachial plexus**, and they serve the arms and hands (see Figure 7.3). This plexus passes down the side of the neck and under the clavicles before heading down the arms and into the upper back. We will note the muscles that most affect the brachial plexus and also how our alignment can impede or clear the way for the brachial plexus in its pathway.

The Muscles of the Scapula

The muscles that move the scapula can be seen to work in pairs, with each muscle in each pair moving the scapula in opposite directions. You can think of the scapula supported in a series of muscular teams. Picture that you have a large piece of cloth and that you are holding it at each end. The scapula is embedded in the middle of the cloth, and one edge of it is taped onto the cloth. When you pull with one hand, the scapula moves that way, and likewise when you pull with the other hand, the scapula moves the opposite way. Like this, the muscular teams of the scapula support it and move it in particular directions.

One team will allow for retraction and protraction, another for elevation and depression, a third for upward and downward tilt.

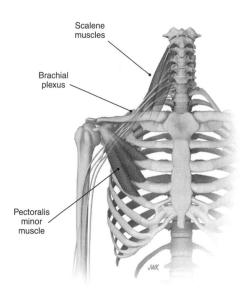

Figure 7.3 Brachial plexus

The teams provide both stability and mobility. Since the trapezius is large, superficial and versatile, participating in all of the teams, we will investigate this muscle first, and then look at each team.

The trapezius

The **trapezius** is a diamond-shaped muscle originating on the lower skull, the nuchal ligament (see Figure 7.18) and the spinal vertebrae all the way down from C7 to T12 (see Figure 7.4). It is so large that we often divide it into three portions to better understand its functions. The top portion comes down from the neck to attach to the lateral third of the clavicle (wrapping around to the front a little), the acromion and the lateral part of the spine of the scapula. Its fibers are oriented at a diagonal moving down

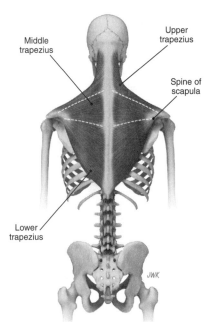

Figure 7.4 *Trapezius muscle*

from the neck to the shoulder. The middle portion attaches to the spine of the scapula, with its fibers oriented horizontally, from the scapula straight over to the spine. The lower portion attaches to the medial part of the spine of the scapula, making its fibers follow a sharp diagonal direction to attach at the lower thoracic spine.

Try this now.
Trace the shape and expanse of the trapezius on a friend. Watch and feel as they contract the entire muscle in a pose like Shalabhasana with their arms out to the sides.

The rhomboid-serratus team
The **rhomboids (major and minor)** are under the middle trapezius, with their fibers running at a slight downward diagonal from

the vertebral spine (C6-T4) to the medial border of the scapula. They retract the scapula in toward the spine, with a little downward rotation of the glenoid fossa in the mix. Their partner in this team is the **serratus anterior**, which attaches to the medial border of the scapula as well, but on the underside next to the ribs (see Figure 7.5). It then wraps laterally around the ribs to attach to ribs 1–9. The serratus anterior protracts the scapula, pulling it away from the spine and around the ribs. (The serratus anterior also comes into play when we rotate the scapula upward to extend the arms overhead. It pulls the lower scapula forward to enable the shoulder socket to lift upward.) The **middle trapezius** is part of this team also, since it is a synergist with the rhomboids (see Figures 7.4 and 7.5). Together, these three muscles

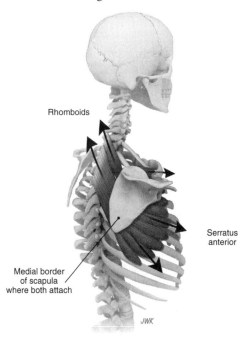

Figure 7.5 *The rhomboid-serratus team: Retraction and protraction of the scapula*

(rhomboids, serratus anterior and middle trapezius) hold the shoulder blade and move it either toward or away from the spine.

Sometimes in yoga we need to highlight the retraction part of this team, and other times the protraction part. Here are some poses that ask for more rhomboid (retraction) and less serratus anterior (protraction): Shalabhasana, Ushtrasana and Virabhadrasana II. Poses that ask for more serratus anterior and less rhomboid include Garudasana, *Pincha Mayurasana* (Peacock Feather Pose), and *Mayurasana* (Peacock Pose).

Are there poses that demand an equal amount from each? Challenging poses like Chaturanga Dandasana, Urdhva Dhanurasana and all arm balances are in this category. The balance of this team is crucial in stabilizing the scapulae on the back so that we can safely bear weight on the arms and avoid injury to the shoulder capsule or the rotator cuff tendons (see below). We want just enough of each—rhomboids and serratus anterior—to be able to lift ourselves up in any of these poses yet keep the shoulders aligned properly to avoid strain of the surrounding soft tissue.

Try this now.

1. Move your scapulae in each direction, retracting your scapulae back and protracting them forward.
2. Put weight on your hands and practice balancing the two extremes of the teamwork.
3. Practice this in Chaturanga Dandasana, in arm balances and in Adho Mukha

Vrksasana. See the next page for more detail regarding Chaturanga Dandasana.

The upper and lower trapezius team

This one is simpler: the upper trapezius lifts the scapula, and the lower trapezius pulls the scapula down (see Figure 7.6). A third muscle, the **levator scapula**, which is under the upper trapezius and assists it, runs from the sides of the C1-4 down to the superior angle of the scapula. Tightness in the levator scapula is a common source of muscle pain, headaches and general stress. In general, our daily tension pulls the scapula up, making the counterbalancing action of the lower trapezius a worthwhile focus during life and during asana. However, some people pull the

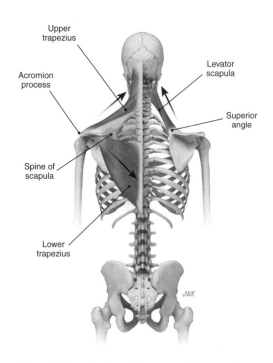

Figure 7.6 *The elevators and depressors of the scapula*

scapula down too much, causing compression in the entire shoulder girdle. As always, we seek the balance of opposites.

Try this now.
Observe this team in poses like Virabhadrasana II, Ushtrasana and Vrkshasana. These poses are examples of three different positions of the arms.

The pectoralis minor and lower trapezius

The **pectoralis minor** is a small and pesky muscle under the **pectoralis major** on the front chest (see Figure 7.7). I say "pesky" because it can change our alignment in undesirable ways while remaining hidden under the bigger pectoralis major. It runs from the coracoid process down onto ribs 3–5. Its action is to pull the scapula forward and down over the top of the ribs, like a roof. When it does this, it compresses the brachial plexus, which passes under it along with the blood vessels supplying the arms (see Figure 7.3). Chronic tension in this muscle can cause referred pain in the arms due to the compression of the nerves, as well as a rounded shoulder posture. You can see the result of an overactive pectoralis minor in a pose like Chaturanga Dandasana when the shoulders drop forward.

The other half of this team, the lower trapezius, pulls the lower scapula back, down and in toward the ribs, tilting the top of the scapula slightly back, in opposition to pectoralis minor. It brings the scapula more vertically onto the back, like a cliff rather than a roof. We need to use it strongly in any poses that

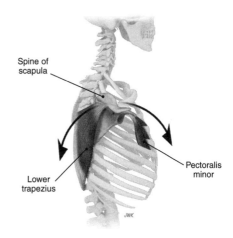

Figure 7.7 *Forward and backward tilt of the scapula: Pectoralis minor and lower trapezius*

are weight bearing on the arms or hands.

Try this now.
Practice Plank, Bhujangasana and Chaturanga Dandasana with awareness of this team. Feel the pectoralis minor working without overriding the lower trapezius.

Now you have met the five scapular muscles (trapezius, rhomboids, serratus anterior, levator scapula and pectoralis minor), and we will proceed to the muscles that move the humerus.

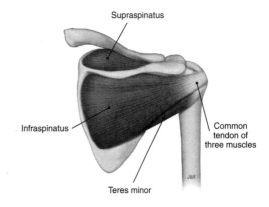

Figure 7.8a *Rotator cuff posterior view*

The Muscles of the Humerus

We'll discuss the humerus muscles in four groups. Beginners to anatomy can focus on group one and group four.

Group One: The Rotator Cuff

As its name implies, this group of muscles secures the humeral head into the socket like a cuff and also rotates it (see Figures 7.8a and 7.8b). It is made up of four muscles, whose acronym (the first letter of each name making a word) is SITS.

- The **supraspinatus** lies along the top of the scapula, in a valley called the **supraspinatus fossa** above the scapular spine. Starting at the medial edge of the scapula it goes along the valley, under the acromion then attaches to the greater tuberosity of the humerus. Its action is abduction of the arm, as in Virabhadrasana II.

- The **infraspinatus** begins at the posterior medial border of the scapula (a bit lower than the supraspinatus) and moves laterally across the surface of the scapula to also attach to the greater tuberosity of the humerus. Its action is lateral rotation of the humerus.

- The **teres minor** is a smaller muscle underneath (deep to) the infraspinatus, beginning at the lateral border of the scapula and also attaching to the greater tuberosity of the humerus. It also rotates the humerus laterally.

Before we meet the fourth member of this team, note that these first three muscles have one large common tendon on the outer edge of the humeral head. This tendon is the most common site of a rotator cuff injury. (See Figure 7.8a)

- The **subscapularis**, as the name implies, is underneath the scapula on its anterior surface. It attaches to the medial border and runs laterally to attach to the lesser tuberosity of the humerus, on the front side of the humeral head. It medially rotates the humeral head.

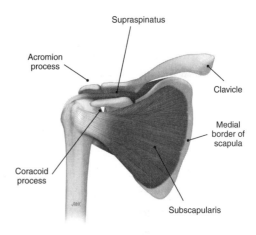

Figure 7.8b *Rotator cuff anterior view*

Try this now.

Find these muscles on a friend, who can be sitting or standing. The descriptions below refer to testing these muscles on the right arm. Note: when you provide resistance, this means that you are pushing the person's arm in the opposite direction from what they are attempting to do.

1. Supraspinatus: Touch the top of their shoulder between their neck and their acromion, on the muscular part where a backpack strap would rest. You will be touching both the upper trapezius on the surface and the supraspinatus underneath it. Have them raise their straight arm to the side, against the resistance of your hand if you wish, and you will feel the supraspinatus contracting.

2. Infraspinatus and teres minor: Have your friend hang their right arm by their side, bend their elbow to 90 degrees, and prepare to swing the lower arm to the right and left, like a door swinging on its hinge. Moving the hand to the right is lateral rotation of the humerus. With one hand, touch the back of the scapula to feel the lateral rotators contract, and with the other hand, give resistance.

3. Subscapularis: This one is harder to find and often very sensitive, but you can touch the edge of it. Just under the armpit, curl your fingers carefully under the edge of the scapula. Have your friend bring their hand across their body, like the door swinging to the left. Give resistance to feel the muscle more easily.

Note: The most common rotator cuff injury is a tear in the common tendon of the first three rotator cuff muscles. Common causes include a sudden and forceful movement, such as throwing a ball or catching yourself from a fall, or gradual wear and tear from doing weight-bearing yoga poses with poor alignment. Yogis need to take special care with Chaturanga Dandasana (see Chaturanga Challenge, page 117) and arm balance poses, supporting enough with the rhomboids to avoid putting pressure on this tendon. People with this injury tend to not want to move the arm, and this immobility can easily cause adhesive capsulitis, or frozen shoulder. Guided therapeutic movement and massage can help to prevent frozen shoulder.

Group Two: Two Small Deep Humerus Muscles

- The **teres major** is a short muscle beginning on the inferior angle of the scapula and attaching just below the lesser tuberosity on the front side of the humerus, wrapping from back to front (see Figure 7.9). Its action is medial rotation, adduction and extension, and it teams with the latissimus dorsi, which is in Group 4. An example of this action is the end of a crawl stroke in swimming, when your hand comes past your side body with the palm facing backward.

- The **coracobrachialis** runs from the coracoid process in the front of the shoulder down onto the front shaft of the humerus just below the attachment of teres major. Its action is flexion and adduction, bringing the arm forward close to the body. It's a synergist with the biceps and anterior deltoid muscles in shoulder flexion, such as lifting your cup of coffee or tea to take a sip (see Figure 7.10).

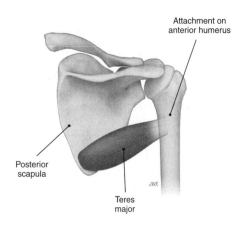

Figure 7.9 *Teres major*

Note that these two muscles (teres major and coracobrachialis) attach to a similar part of the front humerus, which is a common site of pain in yoga practitioners. They both adduct the humerus, pulling it in toward the midline. I theorize that these muscles overwork as a protective strategy when there is any injury or dysfunction in the rotator cuff group or the other scapular teams.

Group Three: Two Long Elbow Muscles

- The **biceps brachii** has two heads, as the name implies. The long head begins on the scapula just above the glenoid fossa, passes over the shoulder joint, and continues down through the bicipital groove and further down to attach to two places distally: the radius bone and a broad band of fascia on the ulna

side of the arm (see Figure 7.10). The short head begins at the coracoid process and runs down the anterior arm to join the long head in its attachments. Both heads are involved in humeral flexion (bringing the arm forward), as well as other actions in the elbow and forearm that we will discuss later. As an interesting note, even though we think of this as an upper arm muscle, it does not attach to the humerus bone, but to the scapula and the lower arm.

- The **triceps brachii** has three heads, only one of which crosses the shoulder joint (see Figure 7.11). That long head attaches to the lateral border of the scapula, just below the glenoid fossa. All three heads join together in a thick tendon at the back of the elbow,

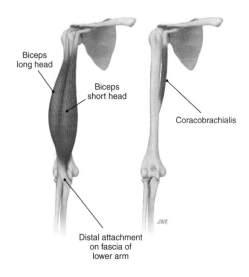

Figure 7.10 *Biceps and coracobrachialis*

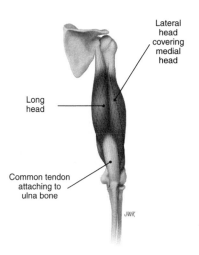

Figure 7.11 Triceps brachii

attaching to the ulna bone. Their combined action is extension of the elbow.

The long head of the triceps is a shoulder extensor, and it has a significant effect on the shoulder in Adho Mukha Shvanasana. When we fire the triceps fully (i.e., by fully straightening the elbows) that long head tips the scapula upward, lifting the acromion away from the common tendon of the rotator cuff. Without that action of straightening the elbows, we could cause wear and tear on that tendon with many repetitions of Adho Mukha Shvanasana.

Try this now.
Feel the triceps and biceps on yourself and on a friend. Especially note their connections into the scapula.

Group Four: Three Large Superficial Arm Muscles

- The **latissimus dorsi** has the largest span of any muscle in the body, from the back of the pelvis up to the upper arm. It has an extremely broad origin: the iliac crest (top pelvic rim) and lumbar fascia, the spinous processes of vertebrae T7-L5, the inferior angle of the scapula and even on ribs 9-12. It narrows into an attachment to the anterior humerus, below the lesser tuberosity. Like the teres major (see above), which is called "lat's little helper," the latissimus dorsi wraps from the back of the body to the front.

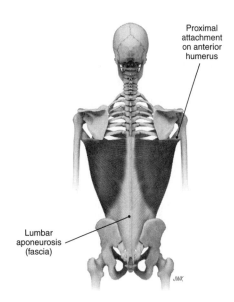

Figure 7.12 Latissimus dorsi muscle

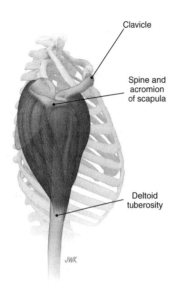

Figure 7.13 *Deltoid muscle*

Its primary action is humeral extension with medial rotation: taking the arm back and turning the arm inward, palm backward. Picture this muscle working in Shalabhasana with palms facing upward. But when the arm is fixed, as in Setu Bandhasana when the arms are on the floor, the latissimus dorsi will lift the torso, which is spinal extension. In Ushtrasana, the latissimus dorsi is both bringing the arms back and helping to arch the spine. We often counteract its medial rotation of the upper arm with added lateral rotation, as in Sarvangasana.

• The **deltoid** is a three-part multitasker muscle similar to the gluteus medius of the hip. Its origin is broad over the top

of the shoulder like an epaulette, on the clavicle, the acromion and the spine of the scapula. Its insertion is on the humerus bone, on a special bump called the deltoid tuberosity, about one-third of the way down the lateral shaft. We refer to the three parts of the muscle as anterior deltoid, middle deltoid and posterior deltoid, each of which has distinct actions.

The front deltoid flexes the arm with some adduction and medial rotation added in (Utkatasana). The middle deltoid abducts the arm, teaming up with the supraspinatus (Virabhadrasana II). The rear deltoid extends the arm with some lateral rotation and adduction added in (Ushtrasana), teaming with triceps and latissimus dorsi.

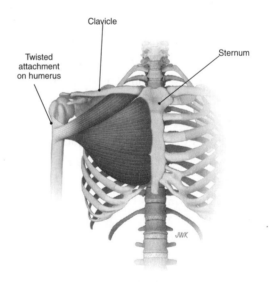

Figure 7.14 *Pectoralis major*

- The **pectoralis major** spans the upper front chest, from the sternum and medial clavicle to the humerus just below the greater tuberosity. Its attachment on the humerus twists: the upper portion of the muscle attaches below and the lower portion attaches above. This unique configuration allows the arm to fully reach upward. The pectoralis major is our major arm adductor, bringing the arm toward the midline, as in a tennis forearm stroke or giving someone a hug. Adduction comes into play in Chaturanga Dandasana but can be overdone. Are you noticing how often I mention that pose in this chapter? It's a commonly misunderstood pose, and I believe that knowing the anatomy of the shoulder can help take it off the list of "riskiest yoga poses." Its challenges are highlighted in a special section below.

In addition, the pectoralis major medially rotates the humerus a bit, and it assists in both raising the arm overhead and bringing it down again. The pectoralis major is important in all arm balances, helping to stabilize the arms as we balance our weight over them, teaming with the serratus anterior in these actions.

From a therapeutic standpoint, the pectoralis major can easily overpower the posterior muscles that draw the humerus back, such as the posterior deltoid and rhomboids. This is especially true since we flex the arms so much in daily life, doing tasks in the front plane. When the pectoralis major is chronically short and tight, the posterior muscles can develop trigger points (pockets of localized tension and soreness) as they try to pull back against the larger pectoralis major.

Try this now.
Find the latissimus dorsi, the deltoid and the pectoralis major on a friend.

Each of these muscles has several actions, so you can experiment to try out each one. Use resistance to feel the contractions more clearly. Then think of many ways in which each of these muscles is working in yoga poses.

The Chaturanga Challenge

Chaturanga Dandasana is a pose that people often do multiple times in an asana practice. Without good awareness and alignment, it can be very damaging to the soft tissue of the shoulder. The most common error is to place the hands too far forward, under the shoulders instead of under the elbows, and to drop the shoulders down, which creates strain on the front of the shoulder capsule and all nearby soft tissue. Optimum alignment of this pose has the elbows bent to 90 degrees, the wrists under the elbows and the shoulders lifted to the same height as the elbows.

Let's look at the biomechanical challenges involved in this pose and where we need strength.

- To support the weight of the upper body, we use the serratus anterior and the pectoralis major, our standard

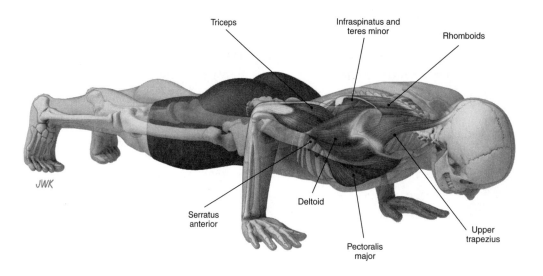

Triceps

Infraspinatus and teres minor

Rhomboids

Serratus anterior

Deltoid

Pectoralis major

Upper trapezius

JWK

Figure 7.15 *Chaturanga Dandasana*

pushing muscles. We're pushing ourselves away from the floor. The risk here is that we overuse these so that the shoulders come too far forward and pull toward the midline. Another result of overuse of these front muscles is a rounded upper back in the pose.

- To keep the shoulders pulling back and staying broad, and the spine in neutral (not curved upward or collapsed downward) we use the rhomboids, middle trapezius, posterior deltoid and infraspinatus/teres minor. These muscles need to be strengthened in order to support the shoulders staying high away from the floor with the hands further back toward the waistline, as the correct placement requires. Yogis often

bring the hands further forward as an instinctive protection—no one wants to do a face-plant!

- To keep the elbows bent at 90 degrees, we use the triceps brachii. Gravity is the opposition for this action, so if we underuse the triceps, we will fall to the floor, and if we overuse them, the upper body will stay very high off the floor (not a bad thing for beginners). In fact, the triceps is more efficient when the elbow is at 90 degrees. When the elbow is bent more than that to a sharper angle, the shoulders drop to the floor, and the triceps is at a disadvantage.

- It's not only the shoulders that need support! We recruit the abdominals (see

Figures 3.3 and 3.4) to lift the mid-torso, the hip flexors and extensors (see Figures 4.5 and 4.6) to lift and align the pelvis, the quadriceps (see Figure 5.9) to lift the knees, and the tibialis anterior (see Figure 6.10) to reach back through the heels.

To build awareness and strength, try this modification: Position yourself with the soles of your feet against a wall, toes tucked under. Place your chest and pelvis on a bolster. Then carefully bend your elbows and place your hands so that your shoulders and elbows are the same height, your wrists are under the elbows, not the shoulders, and your shoulders are supported by the posterior muscles. Then, once you have understood the alignment in this supported position, you can try lifting yourself off the bolster while pushing your feet into the wall. This modification reduces some of the challenge and allows you to understand the pose and build strength.

Note: When you enter Chaturanga Dandasana from Plank Pose or Adho Mukha

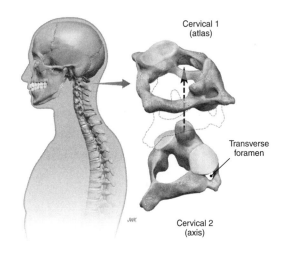

Figure 7.16 *Bones of the neck with insert of C1-2*

Shvanasana, you need to move your chest forward several inches in order to align the arms and shoulders properly. I teach students to take a few small tiptoe steps forward in order to attain this shoulder alignment.

The Bones of the Neck

The neck is made up of seven vertebrae that connect the skull to the trunk of the

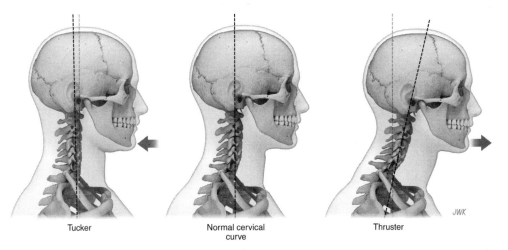

Tucker   Normal cervical curve   Thruster

Figure 7.17 *Neck alignment*

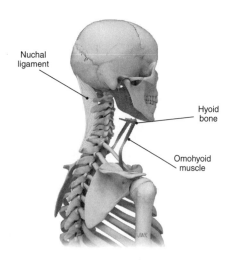

Figure 7.18 *Nuchal ligament and omohyoid muscle*

body (see Figure 7.16). These vertebrae are smaller than the vertebrae below, and they have some special features. While all 24 vertebrae have a central open space (a foramen through which the spinal cord passes), the

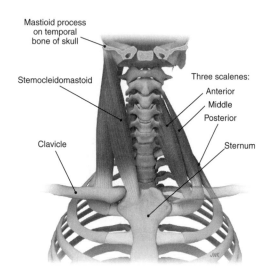

Figure 7.19 *Sternocleidomastoid and scalene muscles*

cervicals also have a transverse foramen on each side. This extra foramen protects blood vessels going to the brain. Its bulk, plus the spatial orientation of the facet joints, limit our potential for side-bending in the neck.

The top two vertebra, C1 and C2, are specialized in shape and function. C1, or the **atlas**, is ring-shaped with no spinous process, which means that we can't feel it from the outside. C2, called the **axis**, has a post, or **dens**, that inserts into the center of C1, allowing for a tremendous range of rotation at this level of the spine. Its spinous process is quite large, so it is the first one we feel at the top of the neck. The dens of C2 is stabilized by a ligamentous collar in the foramen of C1.

C3–C6 are similar to each other in shape. C7 has a much larger spinous process, so it is easy to feel at the base of your neck.

Ideally, the neck has a moderate lordotic curve, concave at the back, but with the head vertically over the rest of the spine (see Figure 7.17). The most common postural deviation from this ideal is for the head to be carried forward, causing a kyphotic curve at the upper thoracic and lower cervical vertebrae, and then an exaggerated lordosis at the middle and upper cervicals, allowing a person's gaze to point straight forward. I call this position the "thruster." This head carriage causes undue strain on the upper back, often resulting in headaches, trigger points throughout the upper back and myofascial pain. Another pattern is the "tucker," as when the head is pulled back, flattening the cervical spine.

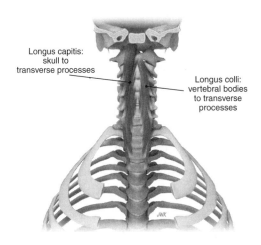

Figure 7.20 *Longus capitis and longus colli muscles*

The Ligaments of the Neck

Each vertebral segment in the neck is supported by small ligaments between each vertebra, as well as longitudinal ligaments inside the spinal canal and the anterior longitudinal ligament going all the way down the front of the spine, attaching to the fronts of the vertebral bodies. (See Figure 2.5) Besides these, there is another specialized ligament at the back of the neck called the **nuchal ligament** (see Figure 7.18). It is oriented sagittally, from front to back like a fin, spanning the distance from the back of the skull to C7. It provides support for the weight of the head, protection from excessive flexion and an attachment for many neck muscles. It is the ligament that is strained in whiplash, when the neck is thrust forward quickly and forcefully.

Try this now.
1. With a friend lying supine, feel the bones and ligaments of the back of the neck with your fingers.
2. See how many vertebrae you can find.

The Muscles of the Neck

A complete list of muscles in the neck is a very long one, so we will select certain key muscles and groups of muscles to discuss here. Beginners can focus on group one.

Group One: The Major Muscles of the Side, Front and Back Neck
The scalenes

The **scalenes** are a set of three muscles at the side of the neck that run from the transverse processes of C2–C7 down to the first two ribs (see Figure 7.19). They participate in any sideward movement of the neck, such

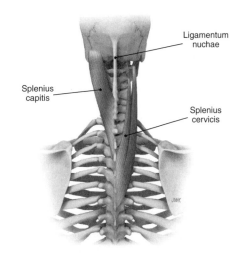

Figure 7.21 *Splenius capitis and splenius cervicis muscles*

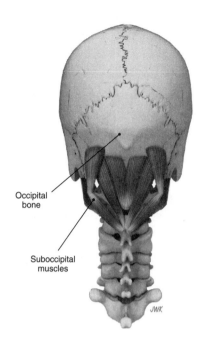

Occipital
bone

Suboccipital
muscles

JWK

Figure 7.22 *The suboccipital muscle group*

as holding the head in standing poses such as Utthita Trikonasana or Parshvakonasana. They also function as accessory breathing muscles, lifting the ribs in forced inhalation such as when you are about to sneeze. The **brachial plexus**, a group of nerves that exits the spinal cord at C5–C7 and goes down the arms, passes under or through this set of muscles (see Figure 7.3). As a result of this proximity, excess tension in the scalenes can cause referred symptoms in the arms or hands.

The sternocleidomastoids

The **sternocleidomastoids** in the front and side of the neck begin behind the ears on the mastoid processes and run down to attach to the clavicles and the sternum in front (see Figure 7.19). Like all muscles that are

oriented at a diagonal, the sternocleidomastoids are involved in twisting. When you turn to the right, your left sternocleidomastoid is contracting, and when you turn to the left, your right one contracts. The sternocleidomastoids participate in flexion and lateral bending, and they also assist in forced inhalation, lifting the clavicles and sternum up. In people with forward head posture, the sternocleidomastoids are very short.

The longus capitis and longus colli

The **longus capitis** and **longus colli** are small muscles on the front of the cervical vertebrae that flex the neck (see Figure 7.20). We retain some tone in these muscles to support the neck and head during deep backbends. They are too deep to palpate.

The splenius capitis and splenius cervicis

The **splenius capitis** and **splenius cervicis** (Latin for "bandage of the head and neck") run at a slight diagonal from the lateral occipital bone to the transverse processes of C3-T6 (see Figure 7.21). Like the semispinalis, the splenius muscles extend the neck and assist in side bending and rotation.

Try this now.

Feel the scalenes and sternocleidomastoids on yourself and on a friend. Experiment with movement that contracts and stretches these muscles.

Group Two: The Suboccipitals

These six very small muscles move the atlas and axis in relation to the skull (see Figure

7.22). They are very sensitive to eye movements and will activate when we move the eyes without moving the head. Eye strain can cause tension headaches that originate here.

Try this now.
Massage these muscles for a friend, and feel them as your friend massages yours.

Group Three: The Hyoid Muscles
The hyoid bone is a small U-shaped bone at the front of the throat that provides a bony base for the tongue muscles. It is one of the few bones in the body that doesn't have any joint connecting it to other bones. There are two groups of muscles attaching to it, some that travel upward, called the suprahyoid muscles, and others that travel down, called the infrahyoid muscles. Their main actions involve swallowing and speaking, but they assist in neck flexion as well. Of particular interest is the omohyoid, which begins at the hyoid bone and travels down and back to attach to the front top border of the scapula (see Figure 7.18). Using this muscle, we can move the sides of the neck back and connect the neck to the scapula, a particularly useful action in backbends to keep the back of the neck long.

Try this now.
In Tadasana, move the sides of your neck back and see if you can feel the connection made by the omohyoid muscle to your scapulae.

Group Four: The Cervical Segments of Spinal and Shoulder Muscles

- The deepest spinal extensors are the **interspinalis** and **intertransversarii**, which span the distance between the vertebral processes from one vertebra to the next (see Figure 2.6).

- The deepest rotators are the **rotatores** (spanning one to two segments) and **multifidus** (spanning two to four segments). Like all rotator muscles, they are oriented at a diagonal, from one spinous process to a transverse process further down (see Figure 2.6).

- The **spinalis** and **longissimus**, parts of the erector spinae group of spinal muscles, have extensions up into the neck that are known as **spinalis cervicis** and **longissimus capitis** and **cervicis**. They extend the neck (see Figure 2.9).

- The **semispinalis capitis** begins at the occipital bone and goes straight down the neck to attach to the transverse processes of C3-T6. This muscle extends the neck and assists in side bending and rotation (see Figure 2.9).

- The **levator scapula** originates at the transverse processes of C1-C4, extending down to the superior angle of the scapula. Though it is considered to be a shoulder muscle, it is part of the neck musculature as well (see Figure 7.6).

- The **upper trapezius** is the most superficial neck muscle. It begins at the occipital bone and the nuchal ligament, then runs down to the lateral border of the spine of the scapula, the acromion and the lateral part of the clavicle. It extends, side bends and rotates the neck (see Figures 7.4 and 7.6).

In studying this area of the body, try not to lose the beauty of the forest (your head and shoulders) as you look at the trees (each joint and muscle). The exercise below will help you to connect the shoulders and neck to the arms and the rest of the body. We have evolved to have an immense movement range in our arms and our head, which requires a complex design. Be patient with yourself as you study; each time you focus on one or another group of muscles, the full picture will continue to emerge.

The Big Picture

To feel the spiraling line of connection from your shoulders through your torso and into the legs, you can do Utkatasana with a twist. Skip this pose if you are pregnant or you have a spinal or shoulder condition for which twisting is contraindicated. Breathe throughout the exercise, and reduce your effort if your breath becomes choppy or strained.

1. Stand with your hips against a wall with your feet hip-width apart, parallel and about 12 inches from the wall.
2. Fold forward to bring your forearms across your knees, holding the opposite knee with each hand.

3. To prepare for the twist, activate your legs muscles and widen your upper thighs. This will bring space and stability to your hips and lower back. Keeping that width, tone and lift your abdominals to support the lumbar spine.
4. Lengthen your entire spine through the crown of your head.
5. Release your right arm and twist your torso to the right, bringing your right hand to your right hip.
6. Press your arm and leg against each other to strongly engage the muscles and fascial lines that spiral around your body. Keep your shoulders as broad as possible. Notice the support and force transmission from your right upper back and shoulders (spinal extensors, triceps and rhomboids) connecting to the oblique abdominals in front, and down into your hips and legs. Notice how both sides of the abdominals are helping your spine to twist (the left external oblique and the right internal oblique).
7. Keep both hips against the wall as you twist.
8. Repeat on the other side.

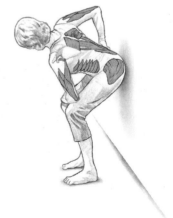

Study Questions

1. What bones are included in the shoulder girdle?

2. Describe some landmarks on the scapula.

3. What is the significance of the brachial plexus?

4. Describe the trapezius muscle. What are its actions?

5. What are the three muscular teams that support the scapula?

6. Describe the rotator cuff, naming the four muscles if you can. What is the most common rotator cuff injury?

7. Describe the pectoralis major, deltoid and latissimus dorsi muscles and how they move the arms.

8. Name the main shoulder muscles of Chaturanga Dandasana and how they balance each other.

9. Describe the sternocleidomastoid, the scalenes, longus colli and the splenius muscles and how each moves the neck.

10. Think of cues you would use to encourage good shoulder and neck alignment in a variety of poses.

11. Design a warm-up practice that will help a stiff new student understand and feel the correct shoulder actions required for Adho Mukha Shvanasana, Plank Pose, Chaturanga Dandasana and Bhujangasana.

CHAPTER 8
THE ELBOWS, WRISTS & HANDS

Think of the many ways you have used your elbows and hands in the last few hours. You may have used them to wash yourself, get dressed, eat or drink, wash dishes or use the computer keyboard. Or perhaps you did something very specialized like tighten the screws in your glasses, play a guitar, sew on a button, speak in sign language, draw a picture or give someone a massage. Or perhaps you've done your daily Adho Mukha Vrksasana. Our dexterity—the skilled and precise use of our hands—is an evolutionary pinnacle that sets us apart from our ancestors. Neurologists say that as human hands developed to use tools over thousands of years, the brain developed to accommodate these new skills; neuroplasticity is one big pay-off of fine motor learning. The hands (and all the joints, muscles, connective tissues and nerves they are made up of) and our brains will continue to evolve as we continue to learn new skills.

The average person doesn't stand on their hands often, but yogis, acrobats and gymnasts do. This chapter will provide an overview of the elbows, wrists and hands, with special emphasis on the demands and requirements for safe weight bearing on the hands in yoga. This part of the body is perhaps the most biomechanically intricate and complex, so we will focus on the big picture and just enough details to help you use your arms and hands wisely in your practice.

The Bones of the Elbow Joint

The **humerus** (Latin for "shoulder") is the upper arm bone, part of the shoulder joint at

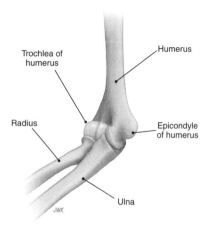

Figure 8.1a Elbow bones lateral view

the upper (superior, proximal) end and the elbow joint at the lower (inferior, distal) end (see Figures 8.1a and 8.1b). It has some significant landmarks that help us understand its functions. At the lower end of the humerus, there are two lateral prominences called the **epicondyles**, one on each side, which you can easily feel. Between the epicondyles is the **trochlea** (still part of the humerus), which means "pulley" in Latin. The trochlea has a rounded shape like a rolling pin, so that the **ulna** bone can roll over it. The bony point of the elbow (easy to feel) is the top part of your ulna bone, and this particular part of it is called the **olecranon process**. It rolls over the trochlea of the humerus to allow us to bend and straighten the elbow. The distal end of the ulna forms the wrist on the little-finger side.

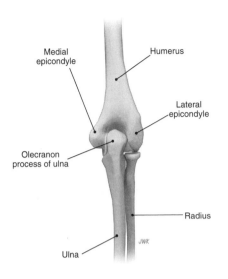

Figure 8.1b *Elbow bones posterior view*

Try this now.

1. Feel your lateral and medial epicondyles and your olecranon process.
2. Hold your arm extended forward, palm facing up, and bend and straighten your elbow.
3. Picture the olecranon process rotating around the trochlea of the humerus.

The third bone of the elbow is the **radius**. Its head is like a round drumhead that fits alongside the ulna, articulating both with the ulna and the humerus at the elbow. When you bend your elbow, the radial head also glides over the **trochlea** of the humerus along with the ulna. But its more impressive movement is rotation, thanks to that drumhead shape. Held in place by a ring-shaped ligament (annular ligament), it rotates so that we can turn our hands upward and downward.

Try this now.

1. Find the humeral epicondyle on the thumb side of your elbow.
2. Just distal to that bump is a small groove, then another bone—that's the head of the radius.
3. Slowly turn your palm up and down, and feel the radial head rotate inside its ligament.

The rotation of the forearm is done by two actions: **supination** and **pronation**. You can distinguish them with this little trick: supination (palm up; see Figure 8.2a) is when you carry a bowl of soup, and pronation (palm down; see Figure 8.2b) is when you pour out the soup. (*S* for "supination" and "soup," and *P* for "pronation" and "pour"). In supination, the ulna and radius are parallel to each other. In pronation, the

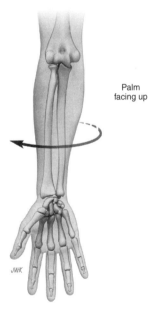

Palm facing up

Figure 8.2a *Supination of the forearm*

radius crosses the ulna, forming an X shape. It's interesting to note that most of the poses in which we bear weight on the hands are done with pronated forearms, with the palms down on the floor. Think of Adho Mukha Shvanasana, Chaturanga Dandasana, Adho Mukha Vrksasana, all arm balance poses, *Shirshasana II* (Headstand) and Pincha Mayurasana. In *Shirshasana 1* (Headstand), the forearms are halfway between supination and pronation, and in Sarvangasana, the forearms are in supination as we support the back body with our hands. Pronation gives us more strength to support the weight of the rest of the body on the hands or forearms.

Another aspect of supination and pronation to note is the effect these movements have on the upper arm. When we supinate,

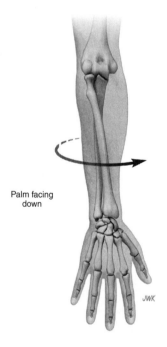

Palm facing down

Figure 8.2b *Pronation of the forearm*

we may also do lateral rotation of the humerus, because of the soft tissue connections all the way up the arm. Similarly, pronation tends to cause medial rotation of the humerus. You might see this in someone who has tight shoulders. When they pronate their forearms to place their hands on the mat for Adho Mukha Shvanasana (as we all do), their shoulders rotate inward. One useful technique to help students understand and separate out lateral rotation of the humerus is to do lateral rotation of the entire arm at first, to "enlarge" the action. Then, keeping the upper arm rotating outward, roll the lower arms inward, turning the palms down. This combination of outer rotation in the upper arm combined with inward rotation of the lower arm is crucial in weight-bearing yoga poses and applicable to all poses.

Try this now.

1. Take your arms to the side, as in Virabhadrasana II.
2. Turn your palms upward, and allow your upper arms to follow that rotation. You'll feel your shoulder blades firm more onto your back, using the rotator cuff muscles and the rhomboids. This is a good action to practice for strengthening the shoulders to bear weight.
3. Keep the upper arms rotating outward and all those shoulder stabilizers still active, and turn your palms down.

You've just combined lateral rotation of the humerus with supination of the forearm;

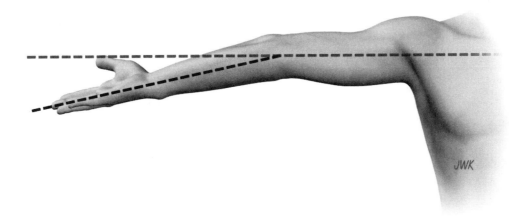

Figure 8.3a *Hyperextension of the elbow*

then you performed pronation of the fore-arms but retained the lateral rotation of the humerus.

There are two common variations of elbow structure: **hyperextension** and **carrying angle elbow**. Both are built in to the structure of the arm, and not the result of misalignment or poor technique. These variations are caused by the particular shape of the bones and possibly the laxity of some of the ligaments and the capsule around the joint. The exercise below will demonstrate each of these variations.

Try this now.

1. Extend one arm forward with your palm up, as if offering something to a friend. If the crease of your elbow is higher than your hand, you have a hyperextended elbow (see Figure 8.3a). In other words, your elbow bends a bit "backwards." This is elbow hyperextension.

2. Now bring that arm next to your side body with the palm forward. If your elbow touches your body but your hand is farther from your body, you have a carrying angle (see Figure 8.3b). You can also see this with your arm extended forward or to the side; the shoulder, elbow and hand will not be all in one line.

These variations can cause extra challenge in weight-bearing poses with straight arms (such as Adho Mukha Vrksasana), since the bones don't form a straight line. You can compensate for this with extra strength in hugging the muscles around the elbow joint, possibly with a very slight bend of the elbows to stimulate more muscle engagement.

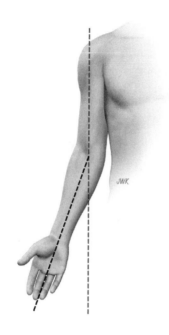

Figure 8.3b Carrying angle of the elbow

The Bones and Joints of the Wrists and Hands

You can feel the length of both forearm bones and follow them from the elbow down to the wrist (see Figure 8.4). On the thumb side, find the radius and follow it from the outer elbow down to the outer wrist bone, which is called the **styloid process** of the radius. Following your ulna bone, go from the point of the elbow (olecranon process) all the way down to the wrist bone on the little-finger side, called the **styloid process** of the ulna. While the ulna bone is larger and more prominent in the elbow, the radius is larger and more prominent at the wrist. But both bones articulate with the next group of bones, the carpals.

The Carpal Tunnel

There are eight **carpal bones**, fitting into a small space (maybe an inch or two long) at the base of your hand. They are arranged in two rows, fitting together like small puzzle pieces, similar to the tarsals in the feet. Distal to them are the metacarpal bones. Four metacarpal bones form the palm, and the fifth forms the base of the thumb.

The carpal bones as a group are shaped in a way that provides a tunnel for the median nerve and several tendons to pass into the hand with some bony protection (see Figures 8.5a and 8.5b). The tunnel is concave on the palm side, and covered by a special ligament called the **transverse carpal ligament** (also called the **flexor retinaculum**), which forms the "floor" of the tunnel. Excessive pressure

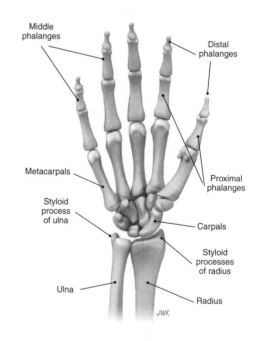

Figure 8.4 Wrist and hand bones

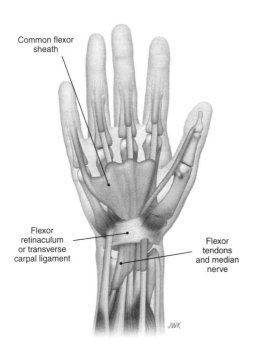

Figure 8.5a *Carpal tunnel palmar view*

on the underside of the wrist can create inflammation inside the tunnel, which then causes nerve impingement, swelling and muscle dysfunction. The thumb, first two fingers and half of the ring finger are supplied by the median nerve, so that is where dysfunction might occur. Certain professions are prone to this problem, such as carpenters, typists, drummers and massage therapists, all of whom use repetitive hand actions and possibly pressure downward through the wrists to do their work. Yogis are prone to this as well, unless we take care to protect the wrists. Later in this chapter we'll address how to protect the carpal tunnel from abuse in weight-bearing poses.

Try this now.

1. To see the relative size of the carpal area and the metacarpal area, make a fist and position your hand as if to hold a walking stick or a ski pole.

2. Flex your wrist, and look at the contour of the back of your hand. You'll see a flat area at the back of your palm; these are the metacarpals. Near the corner of the wrist there is a smaller area with an uneven surface; this is the carpal area.

3. Now grasp an imaginary baseball firmly by bringing the tips of all your fingers together, and you'll see an indentation at the center of your wrist, between the base of the thumb and the base of the little finger. This is the location of the carpal tunnel. The action you are doing is enhancing the transverse arches across your palm, which protect the carpal tunnel when we are weight bearing on our hands.

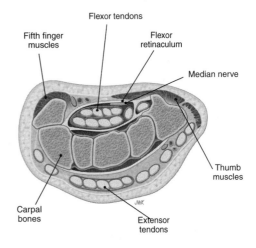

Figure 8.5b *Carpal tunnel cross section*

The fingers are formed by three **phalanges** (the long bones) in each of the first four fingers and two phalanges in the thumb. The main actions of the hinge joints between the phalanges (**distal** and **proximal interphalangeal joints**) are flexion and extension. The joints at the base of each finger (**metacarpophalangeal joints**, or knuckles) are condyloidal; they have flexion and extension, but also a bit of added adduction and abduction. When we spread our fingers apart in Adho Mukha Shvanasana, we use the abduction available at those metacarpophalangeal joints. When we clasp our hands in a bound pose, we are using the adduction available at those joints (see Figure 8.4).

The thumb joint is the most versatile. It can flex, extend, abduct, adduct and oppose the fifth finger, as when you grasped that imaginary baseball. This range of motion is provided by the saddle joint at the base of your thumb (see Figure 1.2).

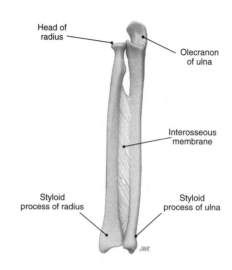

Figure 8.7a Interosseous membrane

Important Connective Tissue

Every moveable joint has ligaments and connective tissue to support it and keep the bones in place. In this area of maximum movement and articulation (54 bones and dozens of joints), here are some of the connective tissues to know:

- The annular ligament is a ring-like structure that holds the head of the radius in place alongside the ulna, just below the elbow (see Figure 8.6).

- The elbow has collateral ligaments just like those of the knee, one on each side (see Figure 8.6). These can be strained by extreme positions such as *Kurmasana* (Turtle Pose), when the legs press down onto the elbows.

- The interosseous membrane between

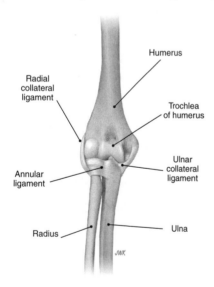

Figure 8.6 Elbow ligaments anterior view

the radius and the ulna connects the two bones all the way along their shafts (see Figure 8.7a). This membrane is stretched by poses like Reverse Namaste (Palms Together Behind the Back) in *Parshvottanasana* (Standing Forward Bend Over One Leg).

- The retinaculum of the wrist is like the same structure in the ankle. It surrounds and contains the tendons of the many muscles and nerves passing over the wrist on both sides (see Figures 8.5.a and 8.12).

- The transverse carpal ligament, which is part of the retinaculum, protects the carpal tunnel (see Figure 8.5a).

- The **palmar aponeurosis** is similar to the plantar fascia in the feet, in that it extends from each finger back to the wrist on the palm side, joining with the fascia that continues up the forearm (see Figure 8.7b). This fascia can become thickened in a condition called Dupuytren's contracture, which makes weight bearing on the hand very difficult.

The Muscles of the Elbow, Wrist and Hand

There are 32 muscles in this part of the body, and we'll divide them into four general groups for easier access. Those just beginning their study are advised to learn groups one and two, then proceed to groups three and four when you're ready.

Group One: The Elbow Flexors and Extensors

The biceps brachii

The **biceps brachii** has two heads on its proximal (top) end, as part of the shoulder joint. Its distal attachment is below the elbow on the little-finger side, on the radius bone and a band of fascia below the elbow (see Figure 7.10). Its actions are elbow flexion and forearm supination.

Try this now.
1. Bend your elbow with your palm facing down, and observe your biceps.
2. Flex again with your palm facing up, and see how much stronger the contraction is as the muscle performs both of its actions together.

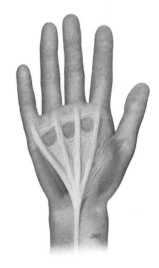

Figure 8.7b *Palmar aponeurosis*

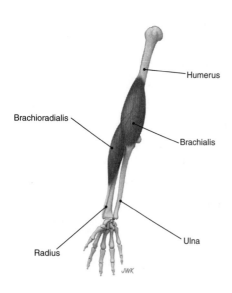

Humerus

Brachioradialis

Brachialis

Ulna

Radius

JWK

Figure 8.8 *Brachialis and brachioradialis muscles*

The brachialis

The **brachialis** is underneath ("deep to") the biceps muscle and also flexes the elbow (see Figure 8.8). It begins about halfway down the humerus, just below the deltoid tuberosity, and attaches to the ulna, on the little-finger side of the forearm.

The brachioradialis

The **brachioradialis** begins on the shaft of the humerus, toward the thumb side (see Figure 8.8). It runs all the way down the forearm to attach to the styloid process of the radius. It is the muscle whose belly forms the rounded contour of the outer forearm. We use it to lift up that morning cup of tea or coffee; it does not supinate or pronate, but flexes the elbow in neutral.

In yoga, we use these three elbow flexors to pull the knees toward the chest in a pose like *Maricyasana* (Sage Maricy Pose), to pull our hands lower on the back in Sarvangasana and to stabilize the elbows when weight bearing on the hands.

The triceps brachii

The **triceps brachii** is the superficial muscle at the back of the arm, starting with its three heads up in the shoulder end and continuing down to attach to the olecranon process (see Figure 7.11).

The triceps muscle is crucial to all yoga poses in which there is weight on the hands. We use it to straighten the elbows in Adho Mukha Shvanasana and Adho Mukha Vrksasana, to keep the elbows bent at 90 degrees in Chaturanga Dandasana, and to push the forearms down in Shirshasana I.

Try this now.

1. Experiment with flexing your elbow, combining flexion with supination (palm up), pronation (palm down), and doing it in a neutral position (palm to the midline) to feel the biceps, brachialis and brachioradialis muscles respectively.

2. Push your hand down into a tabletop or the floor, and feel the triceps engage. Notice how the action of using the triceps to push your hand down will also stabilize your shoulder blades, especially if you take care to widen your front chest and avoid overworking the pectoralis major. In fact, all of the muscles in this group are stabilizers as well as agonists.

Group Two: The Forearm Rotators and Wrist Flexors

The supinator

The **supinator** has a broad origin, including the humerus just above the elbow on the thumb side, the annular ligament, the collateral ligament and the top of the ulna (see Figure 8.9). It then wraps around to attach to the top third of the radius bone in the front. Its action, of course, is to supinate, or turn the palm toward the thumb side, as in Sarvangasana. Other common actions using the supinator are making the hitchhiking gesture and scooping ice cream.

The pronators

The **pronator teres** is near the elbow, extending from the medial condyle of the humerus (little-finger side) to the middle of the radial shaft (see Figure 8.9). Together with the pronator quadratus, it brings the radius across the ulna into pronation. A common pronating action is pouring water from a pitcher. In yoga, we pronate the lower arm when we put our hands on the floor for Adho Mukha Shvanasana or Adho Mukha Vrksasana.

The **pronator quadratus** is near the wrist and is a small square muscle, which gives it good stabilizing power. It attaches to the distal ends of both the ulna and radius.

These two muscles are both very important for stabilizing the wrist and forearm in arm-balance poses. When we press the thumb side of the hand down, we are emphasizing pronation of the lower arm.

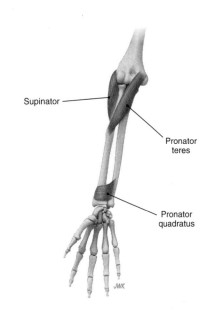

Figure 8.9 *Supinator and two pronators*

The wrist flexors

The following three muscles, all flexors of the wrist, all begin at the common flexor tendon, on the medial epicondyle of the humerus, on the little-finger side (see Figure 8.10).

The **flexor carpi radialis** begins at the medial epicondyle of the humerus, attaches to much of the radius bone, and inserts on the bases of the index and third finger. When we press the thumb side of the hand down in Adho Mukha Shvanasana, we use this muscle.

The **flexor carpi ulnaris** runs from the medial epicondyle of the humerus, attaching along much of the ulna on its way to its insertion on the outer carpal bones and the fifth metacarpal. We use this muscle when we press the little-finger side of the hand down in Adho Mukha Shvanasana.

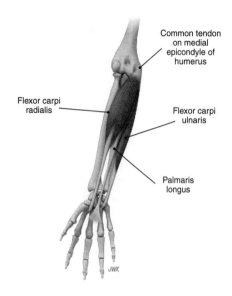

Common tendon
on medial
epicondyle of
humerus

Flexor carpi
radialis

Flexor carpi
ulnaris

Palmaris
longus

JWK

Figure 8.10 *The three wrist flexors*

The **palmaris longus** is a wrist flexor more in the midline than the other two, running from the common flexor tendon to the palmar aponeurosis. It presses the center of the hand down.

Try this now.

1. Place one hand on the floor.
2. Press the outer edge of the hand down, to fire your supinator and your flexor carpi ulnaris.
3. Now press the inner edge down, to fire your pronators and flexor carpi radialis.
4. Press the center of the hand down, to fire the palmaris longus.

Notice how this strong flexion of the wrist with these muscles working together lifts the carpal tunnel a little away from the floor. This team is essential support for Adho Mukha Shvanasana, Adho Mukha Vrksasana, Urdhva Dhanurasana and all arm-balance poses.

Group Three: The Hand Extrinsics

Extrinsic muscles are those with a muscle belly in the forearm and long tendons passing over the wrist into the hands. Because they cross the wrist, their action affects both the fingers and the wrist. This is why we need to activate our fingers to stabilize the wrists in weight-bearing yoga poses. There's a lot of detail here; you can focus on understanding the basic functions represented by each group, and then look at the details of each muscle when you're ready.

The finger flexors

The **finger flexors** push the fingers down in Adho Mukha Shvanasana and other poses with your hands on the floor. There are three extrinsic finger flexors, one for the thumb (flexor pollicis longus) and two for the other four fingers (flexor digitorum superficialis and flexor digitorum profundus) (see Figure 8.11). These tendons all pass through the carpal tunnel.

- The **flexor digitorum superficialis** has a broad origin on the humerus, radius and ulna, and ends at the middle phalanx of each finger (i.e., not all the way to the tip).

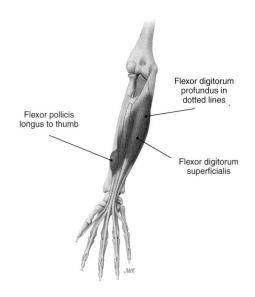

Flexor digitorum profundus in dotted lines

Flexor pollicis longus to thumb

Flexor digitorum superficialis

JWK

Figure 8.11 *Extrinsic finger flexors*

- The **flexor digitorum profundus** has a broad attachment along the shaft of the ulna, and goes all the way to the distal phalanx of each finger (the tip).

- The **flexor pollicis longus** has a broad attachment on the radial shaft and the interosseous membrane, and inserts on the distal phalanx of the thumb.

Try this now.
1. Push your hand down onto the floor.
2. With your other hand, find the common flexor tendon on the little-finger side of your elbow.
3. Press your fingertips down, and feel the contraction change the texture of that tendon. Also notice how pushing down with your finger flexors takes weight out of the wrist. Because those

muscles have long tendons that cross the wrist joint through the carpal tunnel, they will help to lift the wrist away from the floor.
4. As a contrast, lift your fingertips up and feel the weight settle into the wrists.

The wrist extensors

The **wrist extensors** and finger extensors originate from a common tendon on the epicondyle of the humerus on the thumb side (see Figure 8.12). Inflammation of these tendons results in the condition known as **tennis elbow**.

- The **extensor carpi ulnaris** begins at the common tendon above the elbow and runs to the base of the fifth metacarpal bone.

- The **extensor carpi radialis longus** and **brevis** both begin above the elbow and attach to the second and third metacarpal bone respectively.

The finger extensors

The **finger extensors** extend our fingers, bringing a full energetic expression to any pose (see Figure 8.12). These muscles pass under the retinaculum on the back of your wrist, and if they are overused, they will create pressure on the carpal tunnel.

- The **extensor digitorum** begins at the epicondyle of the humerus on the thumb side and runs to the ends of fingers two, three, four and five.

- The **extensor indicis** is just for the index finger, and it is shorter; it runs from the lower part of the ulna onto the tendon of the extensor digitorum.

- The **extensor pollicis longus** and **brevis** are the two thumb extensors, one originating from the ulna and one from the radius. They attach to the distal and proximal phalanges of the thumb.

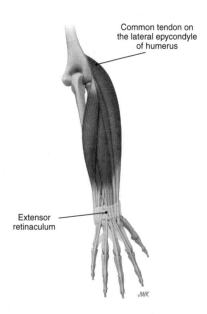

Figure 8.12 *Extrinsic wrist and finger extensors*

Common tendon on the lateral epycondyle of humerus

Extensor retinaculum

JWK

Try this now.

1. Pull your hand back as if you are about to pat someone on the back.
2. With your other hand, find the common extensor tendon just above your elbow on the thumb side. Also notice that when your hand pulls back, there is pressure on the palm side of the wrist.

3. Now do that same action with weight on your hands, as in Adho Mukha Shvanasana. Can you feel the excessive weight come onto your wrist when your fingers lift up? This shows you again the danger of doing Adho Mukha Shvanasana with the fingers lifted. We can stretch the fingers with the extensors, while still pressing them down with the flexors. This is balanced action.

The abductor pollicis longus

The **abductor pollicis longus** originates from the shaft of the ulna and radius and the interosseous membrane, and runs to the base of the thumb (see Figure 8.13). It moves the thumb away from the index finger.

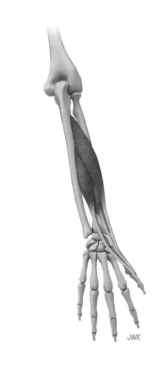

Figure 8.13 *Extrinsic muscles of the thumb*

JWK

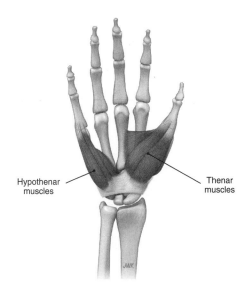

Figure 8.14 Thenar and hypothenar muscles

Group Four: The Hand Intrinsics

We divide these muscles into groups according to their location on the hand, and give you even more anatomical terms to play with. The thenar muscles are near the thumb, hypothenar near the little finger, and palmar muscles on the palm. They are all working when we bear weight on the hands.

The thenar muscles

Use each muscle as directed to feel its action (see Figure 8.14).

- The **flexor pollicis brevis** runs from the flexor retinaculum and a few of the carpal bones to the proximal phalanx of the thumb. Press your thumb into the floor to feel it contract.

- The **abductor pollicis** runs from a few of the carpal bones to the outer edge of the

base of the thumb. Pull your thumb away from the other fingers to feel it contract.

- The **opponens pollicis** runs from the flexor retinaculum to the entire length of the first metacarpal. Pull your thumb toward your little finger to feel it contract. This muscle and the next one form the bulk of the **thenar eminence**, the large mound on that part of your hand. Its strength allows us to grasp objects, and in yoga, to help find our balance when weight bearing on the hands. This muscle performs the clawing action with the hands along with opponens digit minimi, below.

- The **adductor pollicis** has a large origin at the center of the palm, on the middle metacarpals. It attaches to the proximal phalanx of the thumb. To feel it contract, pull your thumb directly toward your index finger, as if holding a yoga belt in a pincer grip between your thumb and index knuckle.

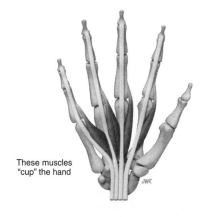

These muscles "cup" the hand

Figure 8.15a Lumbricals

The hypothenar muscles

These three muscles are always being used to help us balance when we place our weight on our hands in any pose (see Figure 8.14). As you read the descriptions, place your hand on the floor and activate each muscle.

- The **abductor digiti minimi** pulls the little finger away from the midline. It runs from the carpal area to the base of the little finger, on the outer edge.

- The **flexor digiti minimi brevis** pushes the little finger into the floor. It runs from the carpal area to the base of the little finger, on the palm side.

- The **opponens digiti minimi** pulls the little finger across the palm to meet the thumb, as in the clawing action. It runs from the flexor retinaculum (at the wrist) to the base of the little finger.

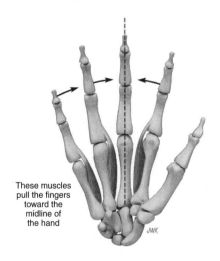

These muscles pull the fingers toward the midline of the hand

JWK

Figure 8.15b *Palmar interossei muscles*

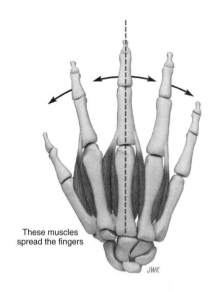

These muscles spread the fingers

JWK

Figure 8.15c *Dorsal interossei muscles*

The palmar muscles

- The **lumbricals** are small muscles between the metacarpals (see Figure 8.15a). They originate on the palm side of the flexor tendons and attach to the dorsal side of the fingers. We use them when we keep our fingers straight but lift the knuckles up. This is the position of cupping the hand with straight fingers, as we might do when we place the fingertips of one hand on the floor in Utthita Trikonasana, for example.

- The **palmar interossei** are between the metacarpal bones on the palm side, attaching to the base of each finger (see Figure 8.15b). They draw the fingers toward the midline. We use them in any clasping pose.

• The **dorsal interossei** are also between the metacarpal bones, more toward the back of the hand (see Figure 8.15c). They attach to the base of each finger and spread the fingers away from the midline of the hand.

Special Notes about Combined Actions

Ulnar and radial deviation are the actions you do when you wave goodbye to someone, moving your hand toward the thumb side, then the little-finger side. You use these actions when performing Wild Thing Pose, moving from Vasishthasana to Urdhva Dhanurasana. They are included here because they are commonly seen as deviations in hand position in Adho Mukha Shvanasana.

Ulnar deviation is the action of turning your hands to the outside edge of your mat in Adho Mukha Shvanasana. It uses many muscles along the ulnar side of your forearm and hand. This action is used to highlight the outer rotation of the humerus, but if overused, could strain the outer wrist if the interosseous membrane is tight. **Radial deviation** is the action of turning your fingertips toward the center of your mat. It is generally not recommended in weight-bearing yoga poses, because it can cause misalignment of the shoulders and excessive strain on the thumb. However, many beginning students will do this until they are instructed otherwise.

The Four Corners of the Hand

The four corners of the hand parallel the four corners of the feet (see Figure 8.16).

Use this sequence to balance the weight on your hands, and to awaken and strengthen muscles that will maintain good alignment in yoga and in daily life. The steps accumulate: maintain step 1 as you do step 2, and so on. Note the resulting muscular feeling of strength and support through the forearm, wrist and hand.

1. Press the inner wrist down. (Muscles used: pronator teres and quadratus and flexor carpi radialis.)
2. Keeping your inner wrist down, press down at the base of the little finger. (Muscles used: flexor carpi ulnaris, flexor digitorum superficialis, opponens digiti minimi and opponens pollicis.)
3. Keeping those two corners down, widen out to the base of the index finger and press it down. (Muscles used:

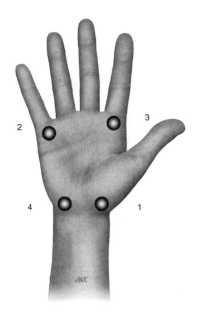

Figure 8.16 *Four corners of the hand*

abductor digiti minimi, dorsal interossei, both pronators, palmaris longus
and flexor digitorum superficialis.)

4. Keeping those three corners down,
press down at the outer wrist. (Muscles
used: flexor carpi ulnaris and supinator)

Preventing Strain and Injury

Repetitive strain injury is becoming more
common as many people spend long hours
at a computer. In repetitive strain injury,
tissues in the arm, wrist and hand become
tight, strained or swollen, causing pain and
dysfunction. Carpal tunnel syndrome is
one type of repetitive strain injury. Yogis are
prone to this condition as well, especially
without careful alignment and warm-up. As
with the rest of the body, moving the hands
and forearms in all directions regularly will
help to keep the joints, muscles and fascia
healthy. Here are a few basic exercises to
practice regularly.

Finger push-ups

Sit at a table with your hands flat, your
shoulders back and your spine long. Push
your fingers down, keeping them extended
but lifting the palms and knuckles off the
table. This strengthens the intrinsic support muscles of the hands and helps to take
weight out of the wrists.

Wrist flexion

Stand or sit with one arm extended forward
in front of you. Turn your palm toward you
while the elbow remains straight. Curl your
fingers in toward the palm, and wrap the
other hand over the back of the first hand to
intensify the curling action. Keep your elbow
straight and your inner elbow crease facing
inward. Hold for about 30 seconds, then
repeat with the other hand. This stretches
the wrist extensor muscles.

Wrist extension

Standing near a table, supinate your forearms
(palms face up) and place the palms of your
hands on the table with the fingers pointing
back toward you. It's like the position of the
hands in Adho Mukha Shvanasana, but in
reverse—the fingers point backward, not
forward. This strongly stretches the wrist
flexors in a supinated position. If this is very
intense for you, you can curl your fingertips
off the edge of the table, or you can try in on
a soft surface like a bed or couch. You can
also do this on your mat before going into
Adho Mukha Shvanasana.

Twisting clasp

Bring the backs of your hands together,
fingers pointing downward. Then cross your
wrists and bring the palms together, clasping your fingers. Swing the hands to the left
and right, as you might do when swinging a
golf club. Then stay on one side and revolve
the hands forward, which will pull on the
wrist and forearm of one hand. Do the same
action to the other side without changing
your clasp, then reverse the clasp and repeat.
This exercise stretches the interosseous membrane between the radius and the ulna, as
well as many of the extrinsic wrist and finger
muscles.

Congratulations! You've been introduced to the extraordinarily intricate structure of the elbows, wrists and hands by which we accomplish so many wonderful actions and tasks with our hands. In yoga, we put special demands on our arms and hands to bear our body weight in a wide variety of shapes. Hopefully, this base of knowledge will inspire you to be aware and to become skillful with your hands while doing Surya Namaskar, inversions and arm-balance poses.

The Big Picture

To feel the fascial connections from your front chest into your arms and hands, try the Wall Pectoral Stretch. Proceed with special care if you have arthritis, any shoulder injury or carpal tunnel syndrome. Remember to breathe fully and easefully as you do the pose.

1. Place your left hand on the wall with your fingers turned backward (remember ulnar deviation?).

2. Lift your front spine as you breathe in, and pull your left outer shoulder blade toward your midline, tucking the bottom of the shoulder blade into the ribs. You are toning the back fascial line of the arm to support a stretch of the fascia in the front.

3. To tone the front line, lift your wrist a little away from the wall and drag the hand forward a bit. Then put the hand flat on the wall again.

4. Now turn your body to the right by taking small steps in place.

5. Keep your left hand firmly pressing the wall, your left shoulder back and your elbow crease facing upward. You'll know when to stop! Feel the stretch all the way

from your sternum to your fingertips, along the pectoralis major, deltoid, biceps and wrist flexors.

6. Repeat on the other side.

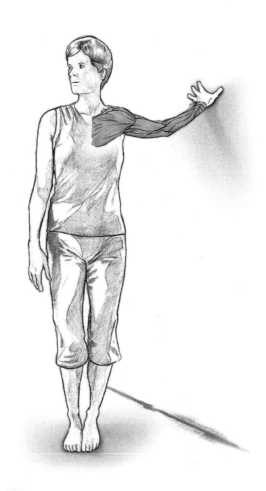

Study Questions

1. What are the three bones of the elbow joint?

2. Explain supination and pronation of the forearm. What is its significance in yoga?

3. Which forearm bone is larger and more functional at the elbow, and which at the wrist?

4. What are the carpal bones? Metacarpals? Phalanges? How many of each do we have?

5. What is the difference between extrinsic and intrinsic muscles of the hands?

6. What is the carpal tunnel? When is it at risk?

7. How can we protect the wrist and carpal tunnel in yoga poses that bear weight on the hands?

8. Devise a warm-up sequence for the wrists and hands.

Resources

Anatomists' Corner (collected articles), by Thomas Myers. Excellent articles that were originally published in massage journals.

Anatomy Trains, by Thomas Myers, Third Edition, 2014. This is Tom's signature work, with material on fascia, embryology and functional anatomy. All of Tom's books are available at www.anatomytrains.com.

Body3 (collected articles), by Thomas Myers. A collection of Tom's articles, all good.

Body Sense, The Science and Practice of Embodied Self-Awareness, by Alan Fogel, 2009. The value of body awareness for mental and physical health, very well written with plenty of research evidence and neuroscience.

Buddha's Brain, by Rick Hanson, 2009. Great information about the brain and practices to make positive changes in functioning.

Fascia, Clinical Applications for Health and Human Performance, by Mark Lindsay, 2008. A chiropractor's view of the importance of fascia in human movement.

Fascia, the Endless Web: Fascial Anatomy and Physical Reality, by R. Louis Schultz and Rosemary Feitis, 1996. Another look at the fascial system as a unifying component of our bodily existence.

Fascia, the Tensional Network of the Human Body, by Robert Schleip, Thomas Findlay, Leon Chaitow and Peter Huijing, 2012. A rich compilation of articles by researchers on the frontiers.

Fascial Release for Structural Balance, by James Earls and Thomas Myers, 2010. Written for bodyworkers but offering plenty of useful information for yogis as well.

A Handbook for Teachers of Yogasana, The Incorporation of Neuroscience, Physiology, and Anatomy into the Practice, by Mel Robin, 2009. A massive book with fabulous information about all functions of the body. Great reference book.

How God Changes Your Brain, by Andrew Newberg and Mark Robert Waldman, 2009. Research on how spiritual experience changes the workings of the brain.

Illustrated Essentials of Musculoskeletal Anatomy, by Kay W. Seig and Sandra P. Adams 1996. A good book for beginners, with clear illustrations of joints and muscles and minimal text.

Making Waves, Irving Dardik and His Superwave Principle, by Roger Lewin, 2005. The story of the man who has worked on heart rate variability inside and outside the medical establishment.

Thieme Atlas of Anatomy, by Michael Schuenke, Erik Schulte and Udo Schumacher, 2006. Excellent illustrations of muscles, joints, nerves, with just enough text. A wonderful reference text.

Trail Guide to the Body: A Hands-On Guide to Locating Muscles, Bones and More, by Andrew Biel, 2010. An excellent guide for learning where the bones and muscles are. Full of interesting details and a sense of humor.

Trail Guide to Movement: Building the Body in Motion, by Andrew Biel, 2015. A fun book teaching all about the movement-related tissues of the body and biomechanics.

Yogabody: Anatomy, Kinesiology, and Asana, by Judith Lasater, 2009. An excellent book that includes suggestions for practice and teaching in each chapter.

Index

Page numbers of illustrations are given in boldface.